COLOR ATLAS OF
MEDICAL
MICROBIOLOGY

SECOND EDITION

Tony Hart MBBS, BSc, PhD, FRCPath, FRCPCH
Professor of Medical Microbiology
Department of Medical Microbiology
University of Liverpool, UK

Paul Shears MD, MRCPath
Senior Lecturer
Department of Medical Microbiology
University of Liverpool and
Liverpool School of Tropical Medicine, UK

Edinburgh London New York Oxford Philadelphia St Louis Sydney Toronto   2004

MOSBY
An imprint of Elsevier Ltd

First edition 1996
Reprinted 2000, 2001
This edition 2004

ISBN 0723433550

British Library Cataloguing in Publication Data
A catalogue record for this book is available from the British Library

Library of Congress Cataloging in Publication Data
A catalog record for this book is available from the Library of Congress

Notice
Medical knowledge is constantly changing. Standard safety precautions must be followed, but as new research and clinical experience broaden our knowledge, changes in treatment and drug therapy may become necessary or appropriate. Readers are advised to check the most current product information provided by the manufacturer of each drug to be administered to verify the recommended dose, the method and duration of administration, and contraindications. It is the responsibility of the practitioner, relying on experience and knowledge of the patient, to determine dosages and the best treatment for each individual patient. Neither the Publisher nor the authors assume any liability for any injury and/or damage to persons or property arising from this publication.
The Publisher

The
Publisher's
policy is to use
paper manufactured
from sustainable forests

Printed in China

COLOR ATLAS OF
MEDICAL
MICROBIOLOGY
SECOND EDITION

Commissioning Editor Alex Stibbe
Project Development Manager Duncan Fraser
Project Manager Susan Stuart
Design Manager Jayne Jones
Illustrator Manager Mick Ruddy
Illustrator Lee Smith

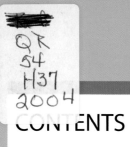

CONTENTS

PREFACE to the second edition

Since the publication of the first edition, we have seen an enormous leap forward in our understanding of microbial pathogenesis with, for example, the discovery of bacterial pathogenicity islands and Type III secretion systems that inject bacterial effectors directly into the host-cell cytoplasm. Alongside this there are growing numbers of new, emerging and re-emerging infections and pathogens (SARS being a recent, high profile example) and so we have added a new section to take account of this. We have revised and updated the text and figures throughout the book and, more specifically, expanded the section on diagnostic bacteriology to include more automated and molecular diagnostic methods. A discussion of biofilms and quorum sensing has also been included.

Our aim is, as before, to provide a framework for understanding medical microbiology and to convey a sense of the excitement of this new age of microbiology.

C A Hart
P Shears
June 2003

PREFACE to the first edition

Medical microbiology is the study of the micro-organisms pathogenic for humans. It encompasses not just the specific diagnosis of infection but also the epidemiology, pathogenesis, treatment and prevention of microbial disease. Although the incidence of microbial disease is not now so great in the developed world, outbreaks of infection still have the capacity to elicit great public concern. In developing countries, microbial disease still exerts a great toll both in terms of morbidity and mortality. It is estimated that there are between 3 and 5 billion cases each year of diarrhoeal disease (which can be due to one of thirty or more pathogens) which result in 5–10 million deaths (primarily in children) each year. However, even diarrhoeal disease pales into insignificance compared with the 12 million deaths annually due to acute respiratory tract infection. Infections such as poliomyelitis, whooping cough and typhoid which have largely been eliminated in developed countries are still important in global terms. There are up to 10^9 cases of infection with polio virus resulting in 10^7 cases of poliomyelitis and 10^4 deaths each year. Tuberculosis was described as 'the captain of all the men of death' in 19th century Europe when it was responsible for an annual mortality rate of 500 per 100,000 population. With improved nutrition, social conditions, appropriate chemotherapy and immunization there was a dramatic decrease in the incidence of tuberculosis. For example in the 1960s and 1970s the incidence showed a decline of 5–10% each year. Unfortunately this plateaued at an incidence of infection in developed countries of 10 per 100,000 population but from 1985 to 1992 the incidence has increased, for example in the USA by 20%.

In addition to the re-emergence of 'old' pathogens such as *Mycobacterium tuberculosis,* with improved technologies, altered lifestyles and improved capacity for maintaining human life, we are seeing the recognition and even emergence of 'new' pathogens. We estimate that over the last 20 years two to three 'new' pathogens have been described each year. Examples include viruses such as the SARS coronavirus and human metapneumovirus (causing respiratory infections), Sin Nombre (causing hantavirus pulmonary syndrome), human immunodeficiency virus (causing AIDS) and astrovirus (causing diarrhoeal disease); bacteria such as *Bartonella henselae* (causing cat scratch fever), *Legionella pneumophila* (causing Legionnaires' disease) and *Tropheryma whippelii* (causing Whipple's disease); and parasites such as *Cryptosporidium parvum* and *Cyclospora cayetanensis* (both causing diarrhoeal disease) and *Strongyloides fullebornii* (causing neonatal death in Papua New Guinea).

It had been expected that with the onset of the antibiotic (or even antiviral) era, most infections would be amenable to treatment with 'magic-bullets'. Although our expectations were realized initially, of late, bacteria resistant to many antibiotics ('super bugs') have now emerged. Examples include strains of *Salmonella typhi* (the agent of typhoid fever) resistant to all first-line antibiotics (cotrimoxazole, ampicillin, chloramphenicol, tetracycline and ciprofloxacin). Most of the genes responsible for this antibiotic resistance are carried on plasmids (extrachromosomal DNA), which are readily transferred between bacterial species and genera. Currently, the emergence of antibiotic resistance is lagging only slightly behind the production of new antibiotics. This is partly due to the misuse of antibiotics and partly due to the infinite capacity of bacteria to mutate, under the selection pressure of antibiotics, and replicate – under optimal conditions they have a doubling time of 20 minutes.

Finally, there has been an explosion of new technologies that have helped our understanding of how micro-organisms cause disease, of how best to diagnose infection and have even defined 'new' pathogens. For example, the hepatitis C virus has never been grown in artificial culture, yet, by a mixture of cloning, insertion into vectors, amplification by polymerase chain reaction and expression of viral genome, diagnostic tools and typing methods have been devised.

The aim of this atlas is to provide a framework for understanding the pathogens (prions, viruses, bacteria, fungi, protozoa and multicellular parasites) that infect humans. Their characteristics, disease associations and specific diagnoses are covered in pictures, tables and flow charts. We hope that we can convey at least some of our enthusiasm for the subject to our readers.

C A Hart
P Shears
April 1996

ACKNOWLEDGMENTS

We gratefully acknowledge the help of Mrs Clare Kelly for typing the manuscript, Mr Brian Getty for photography and electron microscopy, Mr Noel Blundell for diagrams, Mrs Norma Lowe for bacterial culture and photomicrography and Mr John McKeown for fungal cultures. We also thank members of the Department of Medical Microbiology for their willing help.

The following colleagues kindly contributed slides.

Ms L Ashton
Dr R Ashford
Dr W Bailey
Mr B Baker
Dr G Barnish
Dr D Baxby
Professor M Bennett
Dr A Carty
Dr A Caunt
Dr K B Chua
Mr J Corkill
Professor P Craig
Dr D Dance
Dr B Ebrahimi
Dr J Fletcher
Mr M Guy
Ms L Hindle
Dr A Hyatt
Mr K Jones
Professor D Kelly
Professor K McCarthy

Dr I McDicken
Dr T Makin
Dr I Marshall
Dr J Midgely
Dr R Nevin
Dr J Pennington
Professor A Percival
Professor T Rogers
Professor J Saunders
Dr G Sharpe
Dr D Smith
Dr M Taylor
Dr D Theakstone
Dr W Tong
Professor H Townson
Professor S Trees
Dr C Valentine
Dr J Varley
Dr C Wray
Dr S Lewis-Jones

DEDICATION

To Jenny and Anne

Chapter 1

THE SCOPE OF, AND ON, MICROBIOLOGY

■ THE RANGE OF PATHOGENS

The pathogens causing disease in man cover a large spectrum (**1**). At the smallest end are the small self-replicating proteins called prions (*pro*teinaceous *in*fectious agents). These are responsible for the transmissible spongiform encephalopathies such as kuru, Creutzfeld–Jakob disease and, in cattle, 'mad cow' disease (bovine spongiform encephalopathy, or BSE), which has transmitted to humans to cause variant Creutzfeld–Jakob disease. Next in ascending size are the viruses, which range from 20 to 400 nm in diameter. These are obligate intracellular pathogens and are incapable of independent existence. They have various replicative strategies that utilize the host cell's biosynthetic pathways.

Bacteria vary in size from 500 nm to 10–15 μm, different genera having different shapes. *Escherichia coli*, for example, is rod shaped, *Staphylococcus aureus* is spherical and grows to form grape-like clusters, *Streptococcus pyogenes* is also spherical but grows to form long chains of cocci, and *Vibrio cholerae* is comma shaped. Bacteria are prokaryotes in that they have no nucleus but, in most cases, a single loop of chromosomal DNA. Although some bacteria, such as *Chlamydia trachomatis*, are obligate intracellular pathogens, most are able to grow on simple cell-free culture media. Bacteria reproduce by binary fission. Most have a cell wall composed of peptidoglycan.

Fungi are eukaryotes; i.e. they have a nucleus enclosed by a nuclear membrane and a variety of membrane-bound organelles in their cytoplasm. They are larger than bacteria and may aggregate together to produce much larger structures. They reproduce by binary fission, and their cell wall is composed not of peptidoglycan but of chitin. Pathogens in this kingdom include yeasts such as *Candida albicans* or *Cryptococcus neoformans* and more complex mycelium-forming dermatophytes such as *Epidermophyton floccosum*.

Diseases caused by protozoa and multicellular parasites often require specialized centers such as schools of tropical or geographical medicine for their precise diagnosis. Nevertheless, the diagnosis and management of some protozoal and parasitic infections lie within the competence of medical microbiology. Protozoa are unicellular eukaryotic microorganisms that

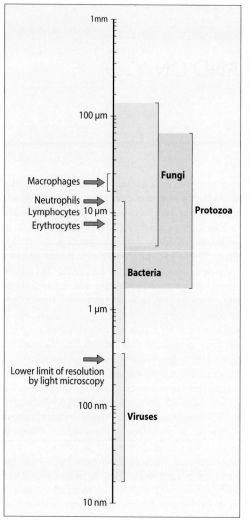

1 Relative sizes of pathogenic microorganisms. The scale is logarithmic, running from 10 nm to 1 mm (10^6 nm). To the right of the scale is the range of sizes for viruses, bacteria, fungi and protozoa. The smallest helminths (*Enterobius vermicularis*: 0.2 mm diameter, 2–5 mm long) are just too large for this scale. To the left of the scale are the sizes of some cells involved in immunity to infection. The light microscope cannot resolve objects smaller than 300 nm; the minimum resolution of the electron microscope is about 0.5 nm.

reproduce by binary fission but may also have a complex life cycle involving various stages and sexual reproduction. They vary in size from 5 to 30 μm in size. Examples include *Entamoeba histolytica*, *Cryptosporidium parvum* and *Giardia intestinalis*, which cause diarrhoeal disease, *Trichomonas vaginalis*, a sexually transmitted pathogen, and *Plasmodium falciparum*, which causes malaria. The multicellular parasites or helminths can vary in size from 5 mm to 3 m long. Some, such as the beef tapeworm *Taenia saginata*, produce asymptomatic infection, others such as the threadworm *Enterobius vermicularis* are mere irritants, whereas *Strongyloides stercoralis* can cause a fatal hyperinfection syndrome.

■ WHAT IS NORMAL?

Although viruses, bacteria and fungi are normally thought of as aggressive microorganisms invading the human body, this does not represent the whole picture. The human body is in fact normally colonized by a very large number of microorganisms that constitute the 'normal flora'. It has been estimated that the adult male or female is less than 10% human. There are approximately 100 million million (10^{14}) cells in the human adult, but only 10 million million (10^{13}) of these are actually human. The remaining 9×10^{13} cells are the bacteria, fungi, protozoa and even arthropods that comprise the normal flora. It has been shown that some 1% of the human genome is made up of complete proviral DNA from endogenous retroviruses. It is thought that they have played an important role in shuttling genes around our chromosomes and acting as promoters. In addition, certain viruses persistently infect humans following primary infection and are excreted for life. Examples include the herpesviruses such as cytomegalovirus, Epstein–Barr virus and human herpesvirus-6, as well as human immunodeficiency virus (HIV). Whether these can also be included as normal flora is a moot point.

In utero, the fetus remains microbiologically sterile. It will acquire microorganisms during passage through the birth canal and from its mother during feeding. The establishment of a stable normal flora takes 2–3 weeks for term breast-fed babies. For premature babies or for those who are bottle-fed, the process is longer, and colonization with aberrant flora can occur.

The normal flora is not distributed uniformly, some areas not normally being colonized (**2**). In these areas, the detection of a microorganism implies infection. Bacteria make up the major part of the normal flora, and anaerobic bacteria tend to predominate at most sites. It is now known that our mitochondria were derived eons ago from obligate intracellular bacteria. Potentially pathogenic bacteria may also be part of the normal flora. For example, *Streptococcus pneumoniae*, *Haemophilus influenzae* and *Neisseria meningitidis*, each of which can cause bacterial meningitis, are found in the throats of a proportion of subjects. Disease occurs when these microorganisms gain access to normally sterile areas. The gastrointestinal tract is the major reservoir of normal flora, and it is estimated that there are some

THE NORMAL MICROBIAL FLORA OF HUMANS		
Areas normally colonized		**Areas normally sterile**
Density of colonization	**Predominant microorganisms**	
Skin: varies from 10 / cm^2 on the hands to 10^5 / cm^2 on the perineum or the face	*Staphylococcus epidermidis, S. aureus*, peptococci, fungi such as *Pityrosporon (Malessezia) ovale*	**Respiratory tract** (below the vocal cords)
Naso-oropharynx: up to 10^9/ml depending on site	Anaerobes outnumber aerobes up to 1000:1 but 20–40% of population carry *Streptococcus pneumoniae*, 40–80% *Haemophilus influenzae*, 10–20% *S. aureus*, 5–20% *Neisseria meningitidis* and 5–10% *S. pyogenes*	**Sinuses and middle ear**
Esophagus and stomach: 10^2–10^3/ml	Usually transients taken in with food. A proportion of adults may have *Helicobacter pylori* asymptomatically present in the stomach	**Pleura and peritoneum**
Small intestine: 10^2–10^3/ml	Usually transients but some *Lactobacillus* spp may be present	**Liver and gall bladder**
Large intestine: 10^{10}–10^{12}/ml	Predominantly anaerobes such as *Bacteroides, Clostridium, Eubacteria* and *Veillonella* spp. *Escherichia coli* (10^7/ml) is the most common aerobic Gram-negative bacterium	**Urinary tract above anterior urethra**
Vagina: 10^8/ml	Predominantly anaerobes and *Lactobacillus* spp. May also contain fecal flora	**Bone, joint, muscle, blood**
Anterior urethra: (about 2.5 cm) 10^2/ cm^2	*S. epidermidis*, lactobacilli, anaerobes, *E. coli*	**Cerebrospinal fluid**

2 Normal microbial flora of humans.

1–2 kg of bacteria in the adult gastrointestinal tract. There are 400–500 different bacterial genera and species that are cultivable, as many again having been detectable only by the application of molecular technologies such as 16S rRNA gene analysis. The great diversity of this microbial population means that its genome, transcriptome and proteome are greater than those of its host, man. Furthermore, it has been estimated that the metabolic activity of the intestinal flora greatly exceeds that of the liver.

Fungi are found less commonly but, for example, *Pityrosporon (Malassezia) ovale* is found on skin and *Candida albicans* in the mouth and vagina. Protozoa such as *Entamoeba coli*, *Endolimax nana* and *Entamoeba dispar* can be found in the intestine in the absence of disease. Infection with cestodes such as *Taenia solium* and *Taenia saginata* is rarely symptomatic, as is that with the whipworm (*Trichuris trichiura*). The arthropod *Demodex follicularum* can, as its name implies, be found in the hair follicles and sebaceous glands of the face.

■ THE SCOPE ON MICROBIOLOGY

In as early as 1546, it was suggested by Fracastoro that invisible organisms caused infection, but until the development of the microscope by van Leeuwenhoek in the seventeenth century, it was not possible to see these 'invisible' organisms. In 1676, van Leeuwenhoek described seeing 'animalcules', which were probably protozoa and even bacteria. It was not, however, until 1876 that a direct link between human infection (anthrax) and bacteria (*Bacillus anthracis*) was proved by Koch. Microbiology developed very rapidly over the subsequent years, but there is no doubt that being able to see the bacteria causing disease was a key event. Viruses were detected and their dimensions indirectly estimated by using very small-pore-sized filters, but until 1933, when Ruska developed the electron microscope, it was not possible to visualize them.

Light Microscopy

The resolving power of a microscope depends upon the wavelength of the incident radiation. Thus, the smallest object visible by light microscopy is 200–300 nm in diameter. Modern microscopes are all compound micro-scopes; i.e. they employ two or more lenses. At its simplest, the image is formed by the objective lens and then further magnified by the eyepiece lens (**3a**). The original light microscopes are called bright-field microscopes because the object is a dark image against a bright background (**3b**). Because the numerical aperture of lenses working in air cannot be greater than 1, the highest objective lens magnification is around ×40. The lens cannot collect sufficient light for magnifications greater than this. To circumvent this problem, colorless liquid (immersion oil) with a greater refractive index than air (similar in fact to that of glass) is placed between the object and the objective lens. This allows objective lenses with a magnification of ×100 to be used. This, together with a ×15 eyepiece, provides a maximum practical magnification for bright-field microscopy of ×1500. Bright-field microscopy is most often used for examining fixed and stained microorganisms (**3b**).

Living, unstained microorganisms can be visualized using either dark-field or phase-contrast microscopy. In dark-field microscopy, a dark-field stop and condenser are used to focus a hollow cone of light on to the specimen (**4a**).

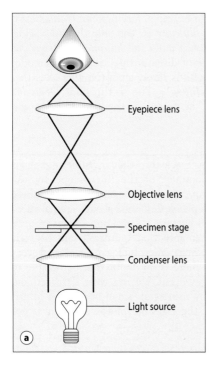

**3 a Light path of a bright-field microscope.
b Silver-stained *Salmonella typhi* showing
flagella.** In the bright-field microscope, the
light (mirror or electric light) is concentrated
at the plane of the specimen by means of a
substage condenser. The objective lens
magnifies the object, forming an enlarged
primary real image. This is further magnified
by the eyepiece. The total magnification is the
magnification of the eyepiece lens multiplied
by the magnification of the objective lens.
Thus, if the objective lens has a ×40
magnification and the eyepiece a ×10
magnification, the total magnification is
400-fold.

Eyepiece lens

Objective lens

Specimen stage

Condenser lens

Light source

a

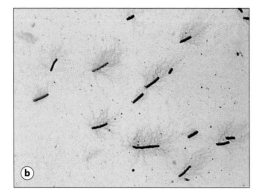

b

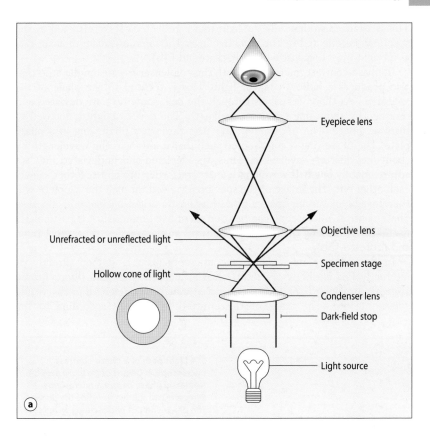

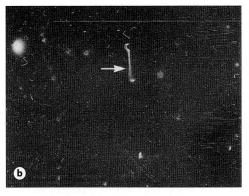

4 a Light path of a dark-field microscope. b *Leptospira canicola*, a tightly coiled spiral bacterium. In dark-field microscopy, only the incident light that is reflected or refracted by the microorganism is collected by the objective lens. The microorganism (arrow) shines out like a beacon against a black background.

This is arranged so that only the light that is reflected off or refracted by the specimen is collected by the objective lens. The microorganism thus appears as a bright object against a black background (**4b**).

In phase-contrast microscopy (**5a**), the condenser has an annular stop that also produces a hollow cone of light. This is focused to the plane of the specimen. As the cone passes through the cell, some rays are deviated and retarded by about one quarter wavelength. The deviated light is focused to form an image. The undeviated rays pass through a phase ring in a phase plate. The phase ring is constructed such that it advances the wavelength by about one quarter wavelength. Thus, the deviated and undeviated rays are approximately one half wavelength apart and, when brought together, cancel each other out. The image of the specimen viewed through the eyepiece will therefore be of varying shades of dark against a bright background. Because phase-contrast microscopy can be used on unfixed material, it is particularly useful for visualizing the internal structures and organelles of bacteria, fungi and protozoa (**5b**).

In fluorescence microscopy, the microorganism is stained directly or indirectly (via antibody or lectin) with a fluorochrome. The fluorochrome absorbs ultraviolet light and re-emits it at a higher wavelength in the visible spectrum (**6a**). The color of the emitted light varies according to the

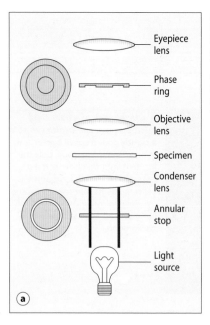

Eyepiece lens

Phase ring

Objective lens

Specimen

Condenser lens

Annular stop

Light source

(a)

5 a Light path of a phase-contrast microscope. b Oocyst of *Isospora belli* by Nomarski phase-contrast microscopy. (Note the two sporocysts inside the oocyst.) The phase-contrast microscope converts small differences in refractive index into differences in light intensity. Nomarski phase-contrast is a more sophisticated method that provides a three-dimensional image.

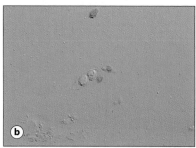

(b)

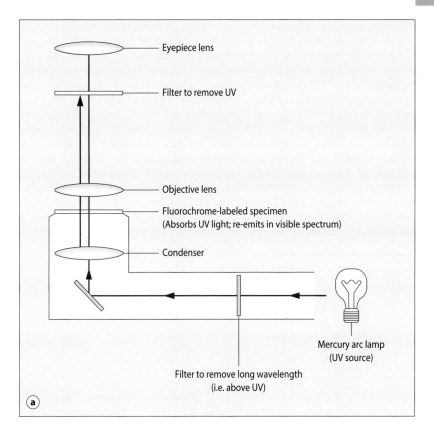

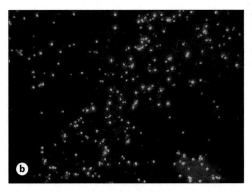

**6 a Fluorescence microscope.
b *Mycobacterium tuberculosis***
stained with auramine phenol and
viewed down a fluorescence
microscope.

fluorochrome used. Fluorescein, for example, absorbs UV light at a wavelength of 495 nm and re-emits it as yellow-green light (wavelength 525 nm).

Direct fluorochrome staining with auramine phenol is used, for example, in the diagnosis of tuberculosis (**6b**). Immunofluorescence employs antibodies to which fluorochromes are covalently attached. The fluorochrome is attached to the Fc portion of the antibody rather than the antigen-binding (Fab) end, so the antibody is still able to bind to its epitope. In direct immunofluorescence, the fluorochrome is attached to the antibody that binds to the microorganism. In indirect immunofluorescence, the fluorochrome is attached to an antibody raised against, for example, human antibody (**7**). Direct immunofluorescence is used to detect specific microorganisms, the specificity being imparted by the antibody. Indirect immunofluorescence can be used to detect specific microorganisms but is most often used to detect antibodies to a particular microorganism present in a patient's serum.

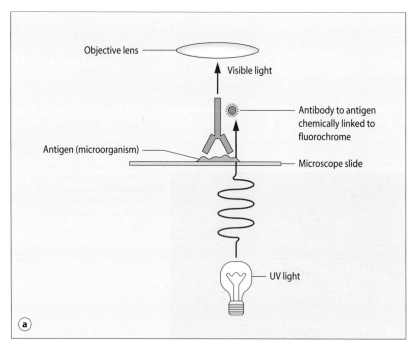

7 a Direct immunofluorescene. In direct immunofluorescence, the object is visualized using a fluorescein-tagged antibody directed against epitopes on the microorganism.

Electron microscopy

Much information has been obtained by light-microscopic examination of microorganisms. However, it soon became apparent that some transmissible agents were too small (i.e. <0.2 μm) to be seen by light microscopy. Electrons behave as light rays and can be focused not by glass lenses but by annular (doughnut-shaped) electromagnets (**8**). The wavelength of electrons is approximately 100 000 times shorter than that of visible light. This means that the conventional electron microscope can resolve objects as close together as 0.5 nm. With the electron microscope, the image is seen when electrons impinge on a cathode ray screen (**9**). In the transmission electron microscope, the specimen is supported on a small copper grid (**10**) and viewed through the interstices of the grid. The specimen must be no more than 100 nm thick and sufficiently well supported and tough to withstand being bombarded by electrons in a high vacuum.

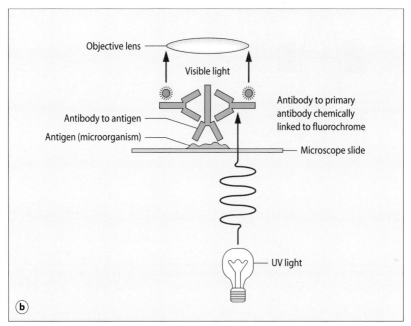

7 b Indirect immunofluorescence. In indirect immunofluorescence, the antiserum directed against the microorganism is added and the slide washed. A fluorescent-labelled antibody directed against the first antibody is then added. This technique can be used to detect either microorganisms or antibodies to the microorganism in a patient's serum.

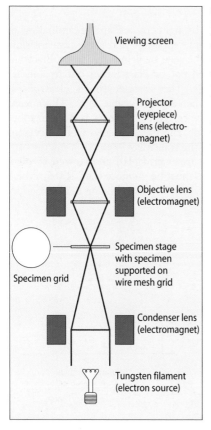

Viewing screen

Projector (eyepiece) lens (electro-magnet)

Objective lens (electromagnet)

Specimen grid

Specimen stage with specimen supported on wire mesh grid

Condenser lens (electromagnet)

Tungsten filament (electron source)

8 Path of the electron beam in an electron microscope. The electron beam is generated from a tungsten filament. The beam is focused on the specimen by a condenser magnet. It is magnified by further objective and projector lens magnets. The electrons impinge on a fluorescent screen to produce the image, or on to a photographic plate for a more permanent record. Because electrons are absorbed by air, the column containing the lenses and the specimen is under a high vacuum.

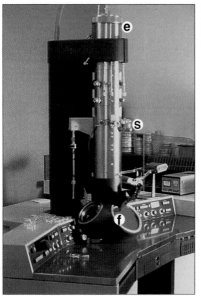

9 Electron microscope. An electron microscope showing the electron gun **(e)** at the top of the column, the specimen stage **(s)** and the fluorescent screen **(f)**.

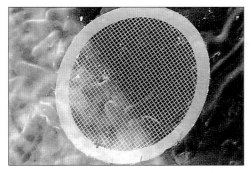

10 Electron microscope grid. This is approximately 4 mm in diameter. The specimen is supported by the grid, and the microorganisms are viewed through the holes of the grid.

Microorganisms may be visualized in a specimen directly following negative-staining using phosphotungstic acid. With this technique, the negative stain sticks around the edge of the bacterium or virus and absorbs the electron beam. The microorganism is thus highlighted against a dark background (11). Another technique is to coat the specimen with a thin film of platinum or other heavy metal. The heavy metal is evaporated from a source and impinges on the specimen at an angle of about 45° so a shadow is cast. This technique is particularly useful for studying bacterial surface appendages such as fimbriae (pili) or flagella (12). Microorganisms or their appendages can also be immunologically labelled for the electron microscope in a manner analogous to immunofluorescence. In this case, the antibody is coupled not to a fluorescent dye but to small, electron-dense gold particles (13). A three-dimensional image can be obtained using a scanning electron microscope (14), although this is rarely used in diagnostic microbiology.

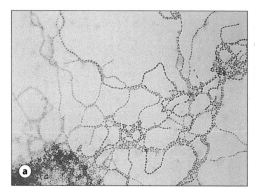

11 a Light micrograph of a chain of Gram-positive *Streptococcus pyogenes*. b A negative-stain electron micrograph of a chain of *Streptococcus pyogenes*. (bar = 2.0 μm)

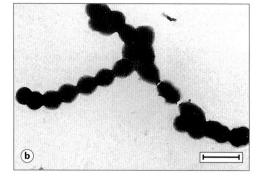

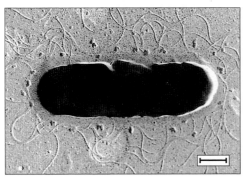

12 Shadow-cast electron micrograph of *Escherichia coli* showing flagella. These are protein spikes used by the bacterium to move in liquid media. *(bar = 0.5 μm)*

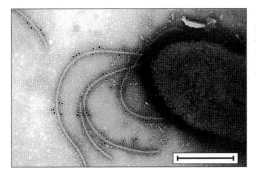

13 Immuno-gold electron micrograph showing *Pseudomonas aeruginosa* flagella. Antibody to flagellin coupled to small gold particles has bound to the flagella. *(bar = 0.5 μm)*

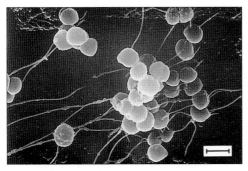

14 Scanning electron micrograph of *Staphylococcus epidermidis*. The strands connecting the spheres or cocci are the condensed remnants of an extracellular matrix that rejoices in the scientific name of slime. *(bar = 1.0 μm)*

Chapter **2**

PRIONS AND TRANSMISSIBLE SPONGIFORM ENCEPHALOPATHIES

The transmissible spongiform encephalopathies (TSEs) are a group of diseases affecting a variety of animal species. These include man (kuru, Creutzfeld–Jakob disease (CJD), variant CJD (vCJD), Gerstmann–Straussler disease), cattle (downers, bovine spongiform encephalopathy), sheep (scrapie) and cats (feline spongiform encephalopathy). All are characterized by subacute degeneration of the brain. Post mortem examination of the brain reveals microcystosis of the neurones and neuropil in the gray matter. This results in a sponge-like (spongiform) appearance of the brain (**15**). There is a gradual loss of neurones and proliferation of astrocytes but no evidence of inflammation of the brain (hence encephalopathy). This is accompanied by an accumulation a fibrillar protein called prion protein (PrP) (**16**). Although some reports have implicated small (10–12 nm diameter) virus-like structures as the agents of TSE, the hypothesis that PrP is a self-replicating protein and the etiological agent of TSEs has gained wide acceptance. PrP has the same amino acid sequence as part of a protein occurring normally in the brain. It has been post-translationally modified so that it can no longer be digested by proteolytic enzymes. It thus accumulates in the brains of affected individuals.

Kuru was transmitted by ritual cannibalism but was limited to one tribal area in Papua New Guinea (the Fore language group). No new cases have

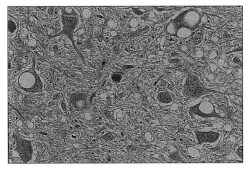

15 Section of brain from a patient with Creutzfeldt–Jakob disease. This showing vacuolation of the neurones and neuropil, resulting in a spongiform appearance.

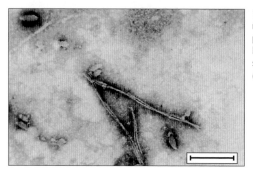

16 Negative-stain electron micrograph of fibrillar prion protein. This accumulates in the brains of subjects with transmissible spongiform encephalopathy. *(bar = 50 nm)*

occurred in those born after a ban on ritual cannibalism. In contrast, CJD has a world-wide distribution. It is a rare disease affecting approximately 1 per million population. Transmission has occurred via stereotactic surgery, corneal transplants and injections of growth hormone derived from human pituitaries. The incubation period is long (1–30 years). The disease progresses inexorably through dementia to death. There is no specific treatment. There are no non-invasive diagnostic tests. Diagnosis is most often made by brain biopsy or at autopsy.

Chapter 3

VIRUSES AND DISEASE

Although it had been known for some time that very small 'filterable' agents were responsible for some infections in man, the 'virus era' did not begin until after 1950. Since then, our knowledge has increased exponentially. This has been made possible by cell and virus culture techniques, by serological characterization and by ever-improving molecular biological techniques.

Viruses are the smallest and most primitive of the conventional infective agents. They differ from most bacteria, fungi and protozoa in being obligate intracellular pathogens. Viruses do not possess the full complement of enzymes (i.e. the machinery) necessary for their replication. They must therefore 'hijack' the host cell's energy stores, nucleotides, amino acids, lipids and biosynthetic systems to reproduce themselves. In fact, most viruses possess factors that switch off the host cell's own biosynthetic processes and divert them into producing new virus particles. This, in part, leads to death of host cells and contributes to the clinical manifestations of the infection. The other major differences between viruses and higher microorganisms are as follows:

- The viral genome is RNA or DNA but never both.
- Bacteria, fungi and protozoa reproduce by binary fission, whereas viruses have a complex mode of disassembly, replication and re-assembly within the host cell.
- Viruses have no cell wall and no cellular organization and are much smaller than the other microorganisms.

Two major consequences of these differences are that, once excreted from the host, the number of virus particles can only decrease. They are unable to multiply in the inanimate environment as bacteria and fungi can. Second, because viruses replicate using host cell systems, designing effective non-toxic antiviral drugs is much more difficult than for antibacterial agents.

■ VIRUS CLASSIFICATION

Viruses were originally classified by disease causation and epidemiological and ecological considerations. Classification is now largely on biophysical, antigenic and, increasingly, molecular biological considerations.

Viruses are subdivided into families, subfamilies and genera on the basis of genome structure and organization, capsid symmetry, viral size, site of assembly and presence and site of acquisition of the lipid envelope. Within the genus, different members are defined by the possession of different antigens (e.g. subdivisions of ECHO and coxsackieviruses), by differences within the genome (e.g. human papillomaviruses) or even by differences in disease manifestations and vectors (e.g. flaviviridae).

Genome

The first major subdivision is on whether the genome is RNA or DNA (**17, 18**). For RNA viruses, the genome can be single stranded (e.g. picornaviridae) or double stranded (e.g. rotavirus); the genome is linear in virtually all (**17**). For some arenaviridae and bunyaviridae, their segmented linear genomes can concatamerize to form loops of single-stranded RNA. The genome may consist of one long strand (e.g. retroviridae) or several segments (e.g. orthomyxoviridae or rotavirus). Finally, the single-stranded genome may be positive sense (can be translated directly to produce viral polypeptides, e.g. coronaviridae), negative sense (must be transcribed to mRNA, e.g. myxoviridae or rhabdoviridae) or even ambisense (e.g. bunyaviridae).

The genome of DNA viruses (**18**) can be double-stranded linear (e.g. herpesviridae) or circular (e.g. adenoviridae). The only single-stranded DNA viruses to infect humans are circoviruses and parvovirus, their genomes being mostly negative sense.

Capsid Symmetry

The capsid is a protein shell that surrounds and protects the viral genome. The individual protein subunits making up the capsid are called capsomers, and the genome plus capsomers is called the nucleocapsid. The capsid can be arranged either in the form of a helix (**19**) or as a three-dimensional structure with three axes of symmetry (cuboidal). In fact, most cuboidal capsids have 20 facets, termed an eicosahedron (Greek, *eicosa* = twenty, *hedron* = side). Finally, some viruses have an undefined (e.g. flaviviridae) or complex (e.g. poxviridae) symmetry.

Lipid Envelope

In general, those viruses which are unenveloped (e.g. rotavirus, picornaviridae, adenoviridae) are able to survive for longer in the inanimate environment than those with a lipid envelope (e.g. myxoviridae, retroviridae, herpesviridae). With the enveloped viruses except poxviridae, loss of the lipid envelope is associated with a loss of infectivity. Enveloped viruses can thus be inactivated by ether or detergents. Enveloped viruses have glycoprotein spikes on their outer surface that mediate attachment to and penetration into the host cell. The envelope can be acquired by virus budding through the nuclear membrane (**20**), into the golgi (e.g. hantavirus) or through the plasma membrane (**21**).

RNA VIRUSES OF MEDICAL IMPORTANCE

	Size (nm)	Envelope	Symmetry[a]	Genome				Site of assembly[b]
				Strand	Sense	Segmented	Size (kb)	
Picornaviridae	28–30	No	E	Single linear	Positive	No	7.2–8.4	C
Enterovirus (polio, coxsackie, ECHO)								
Hepatovirus								
Rhinovirus								
Astroviridae	27–30	No	E	Single linear	Positive	No	7.8	C
Caliciviridae	35–40	No	E	Single linear	Positive	No	8.0	C
Hepatitis E virus	35–40	No	E	Single linear	Positive	No	7.8–8.0	C
Hepatitis D virus	36	No	E	Single circular	Negative	No	1.2	C
Reoviridae	70–80	No	E (double shell)	Double linear	–	Yes (11)	16–21	C
Rotavirus								
Flaviviridae	40–50	Yes	?	Single linear	Positive	No	10	C, G
Yellow fever								
Hepatitis C virus (hepacivirus)								
Togaviridae	60–70	Yes	E	Single linear	Positive	No	12	C, M
Alphavirus								
Rubellavirus								
Coronaviridae	50–160	Yes	H	Single linear	Positive	No	16–21	C, M
Rhabdoviridae	75 × 180	Yes	H	Single linear	Negative	No	13–16	C, M
Retroviridae	80 × 130	Yes	E	Single linear	Positive	No	3.5–9.0	C, M
Oncornavirinae (HTLVI)								
Spumavirinae								
Lentivirinae (HIV 1 & 2)								

[a]H = helical; E = eicosahedral. [b]C = cytoplasm; G = Golgi; M = plasma membrane.

17 RNA viruses of medical importance.

RNA VIRUSES OF MEDICAL IMPORTANCE (Cont'd)

	Size (nm)	Envelope	Symmetry[a]	Strand	Sense	Segmented	Size (kb)	Site of assembly[b]
						Genome		
Arenaviridae Lymphocytic choriomeningitis (LCM) Lassa, Machupo, Junin, Sabia	50–300	Yes	H	Single linear	Negative and ambisense	Yes (2)	10–14	C, G
Bunyaviridae Bunyavirus Nairovirus Phlebovirus Hantavirus	90–120	Yes	H	Single linear	Negative	Yes (3)	13.5–21.0	C, G
Orthomyxoviridae Influenza A, B & C	90–120	Yes	H	Single linear	Negative	Yes (7 or 8)	16–20	C, M
Paramyxoviridae Paramyxovirus (1–4, mumps) Pneumovirus (RSV) Human metapneumovirus Morbillivirus (measles)	150–300	Yes	H	Single linear	Negative	No	16–20	C, M
Filoviridae	80 × 1000	Yes	H	Single linear	Negative	No	12.7	C, M

[a]H = helical; E = eicosahedral. [b]C = cytoplasm; G = Golgi; M = plasma membrane.

17 RNA viruses of medical importance (Cont'd).

DNA VIRUSES OF MEDICAL IMPORTANCE

| | Size (nm) | Envelope | Symmetry | Genome | | | | |
				Strand	Sense	Segmented	Size	Site of capsid assembly[b]
Parvoviridae B19	18–21	No	E	Single linear	Mostly negative	No	5 kb	N
Papovaviridae Polyoma (JC, BK) Papilloma (1–100)	45–55	No	E	Double circular	–	No	5–8 kbp	N
Hepadnaviridae	42	Yes	E	Double circular	–	No	3.2 kbp	N
Adenoviridae (1–49)	70–90	No	E	Double linear	–	No	36–38 kbp	N
Herpesviridae HHV-1[a] (herpes simplex I) HHV-2 (herpes simplex II) HHV-2 (varicella-zoster) HHV-4 (Epstein–Barr) HHV-5 (cytomegalovirus) HHV-6 HHV-7 HHV-8 (Kaposi's sarcoma)	150–200	Yes	E	Double linear	–	No	120–200 kbp	N
Poxviridae Orthopox (smallpox, cowpox) Parapox (orf) Molluscum contagiosum Yatapox, tanapox	350 × 400	Yes[b]	Complex	Double linear		No	130–280 kbp	C

[a]HHV = human herpesvirus. [b]Envelope present but not necessary for infectivity;

18 DNA viruses of medical importance.

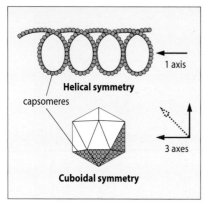

19 Helical and cuboidal symmetry of the virus nucleocapsid.

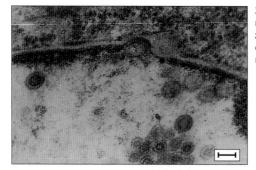

20 Thin-section electron micrograph showing varicella-zoster virus acquiring its lipid envelope by budding through the nuclear membrane. *(bar = 0.1 μm)*

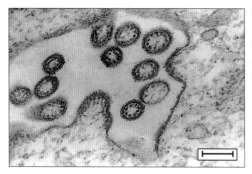

21 Thin-section electron micrograph showing parainfluenza virus acquiring its lipid envelope by budding through the plasma membrane. *(bar = 0.1 μm)*

■ UNENVELOPED RNA VIRUSES

The infections caused by unenveloped RNA viruses are shown in **22**.

INFECTIONS WITH UNENVELOPED RNA VIRUSES					
	Major infections	Less common infections	Vaccine preventable?	Incubation period	Period of infectivity
Picornaviridae Poliovirus	Poliomyelitis, encephalitis	Asymptomatic (90–95%)	Yes	1–35 days	>5 weeks
ECHO	Exanthems, enanthems, meningo-encephalitis, respiratory tract infection, carditis	Asymptomatic (90–95%)	No	1–35 days	1–3 weeks
Coxsackie A	Exanthems, enanthems, conjunctivitis, carditis, respiratory tract infection, meningo-encephalitis	Asymptomatic (90–95%)	No	1–20 days	3–5 weeks
Coxsackie B	Meningo-encephalitis exanthems, pleurodynia, carditis, respiratory tract infection	Asymptomatic (90–95%)	No	1–20 days	3–5 weeks
Hepatovirus	Acute hepatitis	Asymptomatic (50–80%)	Yes	2–6 weeks	1 week before to 1 week after jaundice
Astrovirus	Diarrhea, vomiting		No	2–5 days	7–10 days
Calicivirus	Diarrhea, vomiting		No	2–5 days	6–8 days
Hepatitis E	Acute hepatitis	Asymptomatic	No	25–50 days	7–10 days
Hepatitis D	Fulminant hepatitis (only with HBV co-infection)		No	2–6 months	Lifetime
Rotavirus	Diarrhea, vomiting		No	3–5 days	6–14 days

22 Infections with unenveloped RNA viruses.

Picornaviridae

These are the smallest (20–30 nm) of the RNA viruses (**23**). The name is an acronym for *p*oliovirus, *i*nsensitivity to ether (they have no lipid envelope), *co*xsackievirus, *o*rphan virus, *rhi*novirus and *RNA*. Fortuitously, pico is also a very small unit of measurement (10^{-12}). There are five genera (cardiovirus, aphthovirus, hepatovirus, rhinovirus, enterovirus) but only three – hepatovirus, rhinovirus and enterovirus – are pathogenic for man.

The optimal temperature for primary isolation of rhinoviruses is 33°C, which is similar to temperatures in the upper respiratory tract. Rhinoviruses are a cause of the common cold, sore throats and coryza. There are over 118 different serotypes, and infection with one does not necessarily confer immunity to others. Rhinoviruses are responsible for approximately half of all cases of the common cold.

Enteroviruses are subdivided into poliovirus, echoviruses and coxsackieviruses. More recently discovered members of the genus are all termed enterovirus (from enterovirus 68 onwards). Infections with enteroviruses are generally asymptomatic, and an 'iceberg' phenomenon is apparent in outbreaks. For example, only between 1% and 10% of cases of infection with poliovirus are clinically apparent. The remainder are a silent reservoir to infect others.

There are three poliovirus serotypes (1,2,3) as defined by neutralization tests, with little cross-protection between serotypes. Man is the only natural host, but viruses will grow readily in human and simian cell lines.

Coxsackieviruses are named after a village in New York State. They are divided into groups A (24 serotypes) and B (15 serotypes) on the basis of their pathogenicity for mice. Group A viruses are difficult to grow in tissue culture but will infect suckling mice. Group A viruses are associated with a variety of exanthems (hand, foot and mouth disease) and enanthems (e.g. herpangina), neurological infections and conjunctivitis (A24). Group B viruses are associated with epidemic myalgia (Bornholm disease), meningitis and myocarditis.

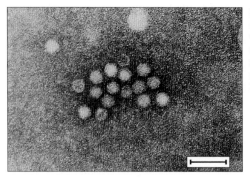

23 Negative-stain electron micrograph of a picornavirus. The virus is unenveloped and has cuboidal symmetry and a single-stranded, positive-sense RNA genome (molecular weight about 2.5×10^6). *(bar = 100 nm)*

Echo is an acronym for *e*nteric *c*ytopathic *h*uman *o*rphan (the latter meaning that there was no specific disease association). Most echoviruses grow readily in human and primate cell lines. Aseptic meningitis, neonatal infections and exanthems are the major disease associations. Enterovirus 68 is associated with respiratory tract infection, enterovirus 70 with acute haemorrhagic conjunctivitis and enterovirus 71 with meningoencephalitis and a polio-like illness.

Hepatitis A virus, which causes epidemics or sporadic cases of hepatitis (**24**), was classified as enterovirus 72 but is now allocated to a separate genus – the hepatoviridae.

The sources and modes of spread of picorna and other viruses are shown in **25**.

Astroviridae
These are small (approximately 27–30 nm), round, non-enveloped viruses with a distinctive star shape to their surface (**26**). There are at least eight serotypes, although serotype 1 predominates in the UK and most parts of the world. It is a cause of infantile diarrhea and vomiting (about 10–12% of cases) and predominates in the winter time in temperate countries. Diagnosis is by electron microscopy, antigen detection or the reverse transcriptase–polymerase chain reaction (RT–PCR).

Caliciviridae
These are also small (35–40 nm), round, non-enveloped viruses. These viruses have never been grown in artificial culture and were first recognized on electron microscopy of diarrheic stool.

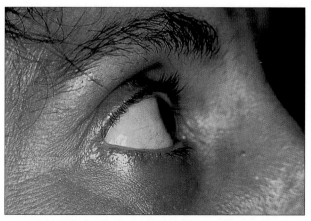

24 A patient with acute infective hepatitis caused by hepatitis A virus.
Note the yellow sclera.

SOURCES AND TRANSMISSION OF VIRUSES

	Man	Other animals	Insect vector	Feco-oral spread	Droplet inhalation	Direct or indirect inoculation into		Nosocomial	Blood to blood	Transplacental spread	Sexual transmission
						Mucosa	Skin				
RNA viruses											
Enteroviruses	+	−	−	+	(+)	(+)	−	+	−	?	(+)
Hepatovirus	+	−	−	+	−	(+)	−	+	(+)	−	+
Rhinovirus	+	−	−	−	(+)	+	−	+	−	−	−
Astrovirus	+	−	−	+	?	−	−	+	−	−	−
Calicivirus	+	−	−	+	?	−	−	+	−	−	−
Hepatitis D	+	−	−	−	+	−	−	(+)	+	−	+
Rotavirus	+	−	−	+	+	−	−	+	−	−	−
Flaviviruses	(+)	+	+	−	−	−	−	−	+	?	?
Hepatitis C	(+)	−	−	−	−	−	−	(+)	+	−	−
Togaviruses	(+)	+	+	−	−	−	−	−	−	−	−
Rubellavirus	+	−	−	−	+	−	−	(+)	−	+	−
Coronavirus	+	+	−	−	(+)	+	−	−	−	−	−
Rabies virus	−	+	−	−	−	+	+[a]	−	−	−	−
Retroviruses	(+)	−	−	−	−	+	−	(+)	+	+	+
Arenaviruses	−	+	−	−	+	−	−	(+)	−	?	(+)
Bunyavirus	−	+	+	−	−	−	+[a]	+	−	−	−
Hantavirus	−	+	−	−	+	−	−	−	−	−	−
Influenza	+	(+)	−	−	+	+	−	+	−	?	−
Parainfluenza and mumps	+	−	−	−	+	+	−	+	−	?	−
Measles	+	−	−	−	+	+	−	+	−	−	−

+ = Major source or route. (+) = Less common source or route. − = Not a source or route. ? = Possible, anecdotal or speculative.
[a]Through skin via animal bite.

SOURCES AND TRANSMISSION OF VIRUSES (Cont'd)

	Man	Other animals	Insect vector	Feco-oral spread	Droplet inhalation	Direct or indirect inoculation into		Nosocomial	Blood to blood	Transplacental spread	Sexual transmission
						Mucosa	Skin				
Respiratory syncytial virus	+	–	–	–	+	+	–	+	–	–	–
Filovirus	(+)	+	–	–	+	–	–	(+)	–	–	–
DNA viruses											
Parvovirus	+	–	–	(+)	+	+	–	–	(+)	+	–
Polyomavirus	+	–	–	–	+	+	–	–	–	–	?
Papillomavirus	+	–	–	–	–	+	+	(+)	–	–	+
Adenovirus	+	–	–	+	+	(+)	–	+	?	–	–
Hepadnavirus	+	–	–	–	–	+	–	+	+	–	+
HHV-1 & 2	+	–	–	–	–	+	+	(+)	–	(+)	+
HHV-3	+	–	–	–	+	+	–	(+)	–	+	–
HHV-4	+	–	–	–	+	+	–	(+)	+	(+)	+
HHV-5	+	–	–	–	–	+	–	–	+	+	+
HHV-6	+	–	–	–	–	?	–	–	?	–	+
HHV-7	+	–	–	–	?	+	–	–	–	?	?
Poxvirus	+	+	–	–	+	+	+	–	–	(+)	–

+ = Major source or route. (+) = Less common source or route. – = Not a source or route. ? = Possible, anecdotal or speculative.
aThrough skin via animal bite.

25 Sources and transmission of viruses (Cont'd).

They were originally termed small, round, structured viruses and small, round, structureless viruses. The small, round, structured viruses have a 'Star of David' surface configuration on their capsid (**27**). This leads to apparent cup-shaped depressions on the surface of the virus (Greek, *calyx* = cup). The application of molecular technologies (RT–PCR and sequencing) has shown that the viruses, which cause predominantly diarrheal disease, form a subfamily called sapoviruses (after Sapporo virus). The small, structureless viruses have a feathery edge and form the Norovirus (after Norwalk virus) subfamily. These cause winter vomiting disease and have been responsible for large outbreaks of vomiting on cruise liners. Finally, it is thought that hepatitis E virus (HEV) is also a calicivirus, although its genomic organization is dissimilar. HEV is a cause of epidemic hepatitis and is spread feco-orally. Diagnosis is by electron microscopy, antigen detection, RT–PCR or, for HEV, by antibody detection.

Reoviridae
Of the three genera (orbiviridae, reoviridae, rotaviridae) in the family, only rotavirus is an important human pathogen. Rotavirus is a medium-sized

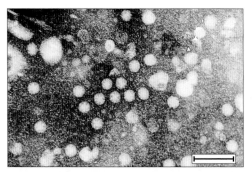

26 Negative-stain electron micrograph of astrovirus. Note the characteristic six-pointed star. The astrovirus is positive-strand RNA (7.8 kb), which is monocistronic. The protopolypeptide is then cleaved by protease to produce the individual structural proteins. *(bar = 100 nm)*

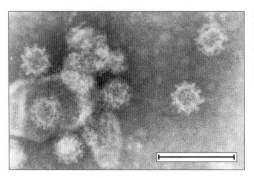

27 Negative-stain electron micrograph of calicivirus. Note the cup-shaped depressions in the viral surface. The genome is positive-strand RNA (8 kb). *(bar = 100 nm)*

(70 nm) virus with a double-shelled capsid that gives the characteristic wheel-shape (Latin, *rota* = wheel) on electron microscopy (**28**). The genome is double-stranded RNA in 11 segments (**29**), and this can be directly detected in faeces of infected individuals. The pattern of migration of the double-stranded RNA segments varies between viruses and can provide epidemiological information. There are seven rotavirus serogroups (A–G), but only group A, and to a lesser extent B and C, infects man. There are 14 G (for glycoprotein) and 20 P (for protease) serotypes expressed on the virion surface, and antibodies to these are neutralizing. Unfortunately, antibody to one serotype does not protect against others. Rotavirus is the major cause of diarrheal disease in children under 5 years of age (20–60% of cases). It too predominates in the winter months in temperate countries. Diagnosis is by electron microscopy, antigen detection or genome detection by RNA electrophoresis or RT–PCR.

■ ENVELOPED RNA VIRUSES

The medically important enveloped RNA viruses and their disease associations are shown in **30**.

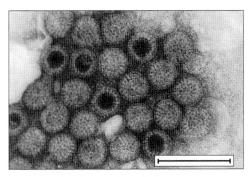

28 Negative-stain electron micrograph of rotavirus. The double-shelled capsid gives the typical wheel shape to the virus. *(bar = 200 nm)*

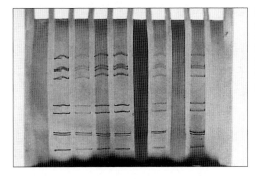

29 Polyacrylamide gel electrophoresis of rotavirus RNA extracted directly from feces. The RNA has been visualized using a silver stain. The migration pattern of the double-stranded RNA provides useful epidemiological information.

INFECTIONS BY ENVELOPED RNA VIRUSES

	Major diseases	Less common diseases	Vaccine preventable	Incubation period	Transmission and period of infectivity
Flaviviridae					
Yellow fever	Viral hemorrhagic fever	Meningoencephalitis	Yes	3–6 days	Mosquito borne (*Aedes*)
Dengue	Viral hemorrhagic fever	Febrile illness (in children)	No	2–7 days	Mosquito borne (*Aedes*)
Japanese B	Encephalitis	Asymptomatic (96–99% of cases)	Yes	4–14 days	Mosquito borne (*Culex*)
St Louis	Encephalitis	Asymptomatic (94–99% of cases)	No	5–21 days	Mosquito borne (*Culex*)
Hepatitis C	Acute and chronic hepatitis	Asymptomatic (20–40%)	No	40 days	6 months to lifetime
Togaviridae					
Eastern equine	Encephalitis	Asymptomatic (88–97%)	No	5–15 days	Mosquito borne (*Aedes*)
Chikungunya	Fever, rash, polyarthritis	–	No	1–6 days	Mosquito borne (*Aedes*)
Rubella	German measles	Asymptomatic (80–90%)	Yes	16–21 days	1 week before, 3 weeks after rash
Coronavirus	Common cold	Pneumonia, diarrhea	No	3 days	1 week
SARS coronavirus	Severe acute respiratory syndrome	Diarrhea	No	6–10 days	2–3 weeks
Rabies	Encephalitis (>99% mortality)		Yes	9 days to years depending on site of inoculation	Until death, but no case of human-to-human transmission
Retroviridae					
HTLV1	Tropical spastic paresis	Adult T-cell leukemia, asymptomatic (90–99%)	No	3 weeks to 15 years	Lifetime
HIV (1 and 2)	AIDS	Meningoencephalitis, asymptomatic	No	2–6 months (infants) 4–15 years (adults)	Lifetime
Arenaviridae					
LCM	Febrile illness	Aseptic meningitis, asymptomatic (95%)	No	7–21 days	?
Lassa, Junin, Machupo, Sabia	Hemorrhagic fever	'Flu-like' illness, asymptomatic (20–30%)	No	10–11 days	?

INFECTIONS BY ENVELOPED RNA VIRUSES (Cont'd)					
	Major diseases	Less common diseases	Vaccine preventable	Incubation period	Transmission and period of infectivity
Bunyaviridae					
Bunyamwera	Encephalitis	Myalgia, fever	No	3–7 days	Mosquito borne
Phlebovirus	Sandfly fever, encephalitis	Asymptomatic (25%)	No	3–7 days	Mosquito or sandfly borne
Nairovirus	Hemorrhagic fever	'Flu-like' illness	No	3–12 days	Tick borne
Hantavirus	Hemorrhagic fever/pneumonia	Asymptomatic (30–95%)	No	1–6 weeks	No person-to-person spread
Myxoviridae					
Influenza A, B, C	Influenza	Encephalitis	Yes	1–3 days	1–2 weeks
Paramyxoviridae					
Parainfluenza	Laryngo-tracheobronchitis	Croup in infants	No	1–3 days	1–2 weeks
Mumps	Parotitis	Aseptic meningitis	Yes	12–25 days	7 days pre and 15 days post parotitis
Measles	Acute exanthem	Pneumonia, encephalitis	Yes	10–14 days	4 days pre rash until desquamation
Respiratory syncytial virus	Bronchiolitis	Pneumonia	No	3–7 days	2–3 weeks
Human metapneumovirus	Bronchiolitis	Pneumonia	No	3–7 days	2–3 weeks
Filoviridae					
Marburg, Ebola	Hemorrhagic fever (90% mortality)	–	No	7–9 days	4–5 weeks

30 Infections by enveloped RNA viruses.

The term arboviruses was a classification used for those viruses that were transmitted to man by biting insects (*ar*thropod *bo*rne). Such viruses multiply in the insect vector and are injected into man when the insect next feeds. This grouping was based on ecological considerations, and arboviruses in fact comprise several virus families including togaviridae, flaviviridae and bunyaviridae.

Flaviviridae

These are small (40–50 nm), enveloped viruses with a single-stranded, positive-sense RNA genome (of approximately 10 kb). The symmetry of their capsid is undefined. Many have the mosquito as the vector and cause viral hemorrhagic fever (yellow fever and dengue viruses) and meningo-encephalitis (Japanese encephalitis and St Louis viruses). Diagnosis is by virus isolation (which requires special containment facilities) or the detection of an antibody response.

Hepatitis C virus is related to the flaviviridae but is now included in a separate family, the hepaciviridae. It has no insect vector. It is an important cause of parenterally acquired non-hepatitis B hepatitis (approximately 90% of cases). Infection is transmitted from blood to blood by transfusion, transplantation, needle-stick injury or the sharing of needles by intravenous drug abusers. It produces chronic hepatitis, and the virus may persist for life in the liver. Diagnosis is by the detection of specific antibody or the RT–PCR detection of viral genome.

Togaviridae

The alphaviruses and rubiviruses, and possibly pestiviruses, are the genera that are pathogenic for man (**31**). The alphaviruses are transmitted principally via mosquitoes and cause encephalitis (e.g. Eastern equine encephalitis virus) or a febrile exanthem with polyarthritis (e.g. chikungunya). All have a single-stranded, linear, positive-sense RNA genome

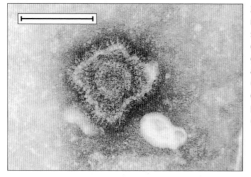

31 Negative-stain electron micrograph of a togavirus. The spherical, enveloped virion has a diameter of 60–70 nm with glycoprotein spikes on the surface and an eicosahedral nucleocapsid (approximately 25–35 nm in diameter). It has a single, linear, positive-sense genome (12 kb). *(bar = 70 nm)*

(of about 12 kb). Viruses replicate within the cytoplasm and release by budding. Diagnosis is by serology and/or virus isolation.

Rubellavirus is the only member of the genus rubivirus. It is transmitted by contact and the airborne route, and causes a febrile childhood exanthem, although in many cases the infection is asymptomatic. It causes most problems if infection occurs during pregnancy. Rubellavirus can cross the placenta to infect the fetus, causing intrauterine death (an 80% risk during the first trimester) or congenital malformations.

The pestiviruses cause diarrheal disease in cattle (bovine diarrheal virus) and pigs (European swine fever). There are recent reports linking a pestivirus to human diarrheal disease.

Arenaviridae

These are pleomorphic enveloped RNA viruses varying in size from 50 to 300 nm in diameter. The virus contains electron-dense granules rich in RNA that resemble ribosomes (**32**) and give the appearance of grains of sand (Greek, *arena* = grain of sand). The genome consists of two single strands of positive or ambisense RNA. These can be linear or join to form a loop.

Infections are zoonotic. The various arenaviruses asymptomatically and persistently infect different rodent species, man being infected through contact with their excreta. Lymphocytic choriomeningitis virus is the only arenavirus found in Europe. It is excreted in mouse (*Mus musculus*) urine and is a rare cause of aseptic meningitis. The remaining arenaviruses are causes of viral hemorrhagic fever. In West Africa, Lassa fever virus persistently infects the multimammate rat (*Mastomys natalensis*) and is excreted in its urine. Inhalation or ingestion of the urine can result in infection, which can range from being asymptomatic through pharyngitis and fever to full-blown hemorrhagic fever with bleeding into the skin and viscera. Person-to-person transmission cannot be ruled out. The South American hemorrhagic fever viruses – Junin (in Argentina), Machupo (in Bolivia), Guanarito (in

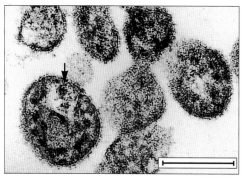

32 Thin-section electron micrograph of an arenavirus. The virus is a spherical, enveloped RNA virus with a largely positive-sense genome. The electron-dense granules (arrow) are ribosomes. *(bar = 200 nm)*

Venezuela) and Sabia (in Brazil) – persistently infect *Calomys* spp (vesper mouse). They produce a similar clinical picture to Lassa fever. Recently, Whitewater Arroyo virus, which persistently infects *Neotoma albigula*, has emerged as a cause of viral hemorrhagic fever in California, USA.

Bunyaviridae

This is a large family of viruses some of which are transmitted by insects (bunyamwera, nairo and phleboviruses), some infect plants (tospovirus) and some are zoonotic (hantaviruses). All, however, are spherical (95 nm), enveloped viruses (**33**) with a cuboidal nucleocapsid. Their RNA genome is linear in three segments and is mostly negative sense, although some are ambisense. The bunyamwera viruses are found world-wide, are transmitted by mosquitoes and may cause encephalitis (e.g. LaCrosse), fever with myalgia (e.g. Guama) or undifferentiated febrile illness (e.g. Tahnya). There are approximately 45 phleboviruses but not all cause disease in man. Sandfly fever is transmitted by phlebotomine flies and is a febrile illness with headache, photophobia and joint pains. The disease is self-limiting and recovery complete, no deaths having been recorded. Nairoviruses are transmitted by ticks, the most important disease being Congo-Crimean hemorrhagic fever. It may also be transmitted person-to-person. Finally, the hantaviruses persistently infect a variety of animal species (predominantly rodents) and are excreted in their urine and saliva. Two distinct clinical syndromes occur. Hemorrhagic fever with renal syndrome (HFRS) occurs throughout the world. Severe HFRS occurs in the Far East (Hantaan) and the Balkans (Fojnica, Porogia), moderate HFRS (Seoul) occurs throughout the world, and mild HFRS (nephropathia epidemica) caused by Puumala virus occurs in northern Europe. The recently described hantavirus pulmonary syndrome is the result of Sin Nombre and numerous other (e.g. Andes, Bayou) viruses, and cases have occurred with high mortality (around 60%) throughout North, Central and South America.

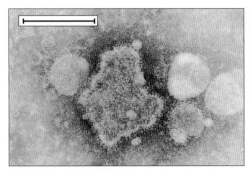

33 Negative-stain electron micrograph of Puumala virus. This is a hantavirus in the family Bunyaviridae. It is an enveloped virus with a cuboidal, ambisense RNA genome. The envelope has a tessellated appearance.
(bar = 100 nm)

The diagnosis of each of the above infections is by serology, antigen detection, culture or RT–PCR. They require special containment facilities.

Filoviridae

These are enveloped viruses with a helical nucleocapsid. They form rod-like or even branching structures (**34**) up to 14 μm long and 80 nm in diameter. They cause hemorrhagic fever with a high case-fatality rate (90%). They are zoonotic, but person-to-person spread also occurs through either body secretions (saliva, sputum) or blood. Monkeys can transmit infection to man, the first human cases in Germany (Marburg) in 1967 being acquired in this fashion, but the primary reservoir of infection is unclear. Since 1976, numerous outbreaks of infection have occurred in northern Zaire (Ebola), southern Sudan, central Zaire (in 1995) and most recently northern Uganda (2000).

Rhabdoviridae

Rabies virus is the major human pathogen here. It is a bullet-shaped, enveloped virus with a helical nucleocapsid (**35**). It has a single-stranded, negative-sense genome (13–16 kb). The genus is called lyssavirus (Greek,

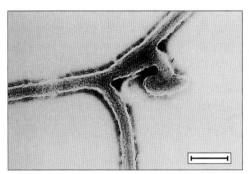

34 Negative-stain electron micrograph of Ebola virus, a member of the Filoviridae. This is a filamentous, occasionally branching, enveloped virus with a helical RNA genome. *(bar = 200 nm)*

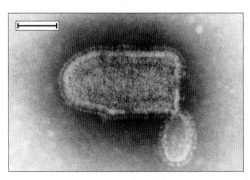

35 Negative-stain electron micrograph of rabies virus. This is a bullet-shaped, enveloped virus with a helical, negative-sense RNA genome. *(bar = 50 nm)*

lyssa = rage). Rabies is a zoonotic infection, the greatest risk of transmission being from adult unvaccinated dogs. Infection has also been transmitted from vampire bats, foxes, cats, raccoons and jackals. Infection is usually acquired by bites but can also be via the inoculation of saliva into open cuts or even on to mucous membranes. The virus ascends via the peripheral nerves to the brain. The incubation period varies according to the distance of the site of inoculation from the brain: it can be as short as 9 days and as long as 3 years. Cases of human rabies caused by other lyssaviruses, including Australian and European bat lyssaviruses, have recently occurred following bat bites.

Coronaviridae

Coronaviruses are pleomorphic, enveloped, helical viruses with club-shaped glycoprotein spikes on their surface (**36**). There are two groups of anti-genically related strains of human coronavirus. Coronaviruses are a cause of the common cold and responsible for 5–15% of cases of upper respiratory tract infection in children and adults. They may also be a cause of diarrheal disease. In 2002, cases of severe acute respiratory syndrome (SARS) emerged in Guangdong, China, and spread world-wide. A new coronavirus (SARS-Cov) was found to be the cause.

Orthomyxoviridae

The influenza viruses are enveloped RNA viruses with a helical nucleocapsid and a segmented, single-stranded, negative-sense, linear genome (**37**). There are three distinct influenza viruses (A, B, C), based on antigens on the nucleoprotein.

There is a fringe of glycoprotein spikes on the surface of the virus that mediates attachment to and penetration into the host cell (hemagglutinin) and the release of progeny virus (neuraminidase). Antibodies to these spikes provide protective immunity, and subunit vaccines employing purified hemagglutinin and neuraminidase spikes are used to induce immunity (**38**).

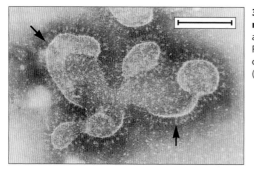

36 Negative-stain electron micrograph of coronavirus. This is an enveloped, pleomorphic, helical RNA virus. Note the characteristic club-shaped glycoprotein spikes (arrows). *(bar = 50 nm)*

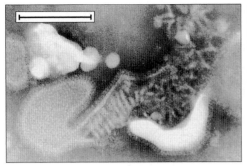

37 Negative-stain electron micrograph of influenza virus. This is an enveloped, helical virus with a linear, segmented, negative-sense RNA genome. There are two types of glycoprotein spike on the surface that mediate hemagglutinin and neuraminidase activities. *(bar = 100 nm)*

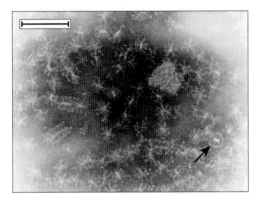

38 Negative-stain electron micrograph of hemagglutinin and neuraminidase glycoproteins. These have been prepared from whole influenza virus by detergent solubilization of the envelope and separated from the nucleocapsid by centrifugation. The hemagglutinins assume star-shaped figures and the neuraminidase cartwheels (arrow). They are used in a subunit vaccine to prevent influenza. *(bar = 50 nm)*

Unfortunately, the antigenic structure of the hemagglutinins, and to a lesser extent neuraminidase, of group A influenza viruses can vary. This occurs in two ways: antigenic drift and antigenic shift. Antigenic shift is a slow change resulting from a gradual accumulation of nucleotide substitutions in the HA gene, resulting in an approximate annual change in amino acid composition of 1%. This is responsible for the epidemics of influenza that affect a proportion of the population each winter. Antigenic shift is a major change resulting from recombinations between different influenza viruses. This results in a virus with a 'new' antigenic HA and a pandemic that affects populations throughout the world.

Paramyxoviridae

The paramyxoviridae are also enveloped viruses with a helical nucleocapsid (**39**). They differ from orthomyxoviruses in having an unsegmented RNA genome. There are three major genera that are pathogenic for man: parainfluenza, morbilli- and pneumoviridae. The parainfluenza viruses (1, 2,

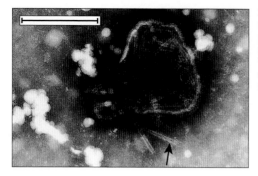

39 Negative-stain electron micrograph of measles virus (a paramyxovirus). The lipid envelope has burst, and the typical 'herring-bone' (arrow) appearance of the helical nucleocapsid can be seen. *(bar = 100 nm)*

3, 4a, 4b) cause respiratory tract infections and, in infants, croup. The other member of the genus, mumps virus, causes the acute childhood infectious disease, characterized by parotitis and occasionally oophoritis, orchitis, pancreatitis and aseptic meningitis.

Measles virus is the human morbillivirus, canine distemper virus infecting dogs and rinderpest cattle. Measles is an acute febrile exanthematous disease of childhood, which, in developing countries, has a dire effect. The diagnosis of ortho- and paramyxoviruses can be by immunofluorescent antigen test, virus culture, RT–PCR or serology.

Retroviridae

This is a large family of enveloped viruses with a cuboidal nucleocapsid (**40**). Each nucleocapsid contains two copies of a linear, positive-sense, single-stranded RNA genome (3.5–9.0 kb). These viruses have the ability to turn the RNA genome back (Greek, *retros* = backwards) to a double-stranded DNA provirus, which then becomes integrated into the genome of the host cell. This is mediated by gene products in the *pol* region (**41**), including reverse transcriptase, endonuclease and integrase.

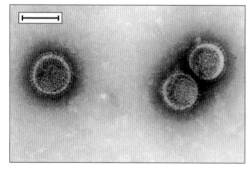

40 Negative-stain electron micrograph of human immunodeficiency virus (a retrovirus). The glycoprotein spikes (composed of three molecules each of gp120 and gp41) can be seen on the surface. The virus has a cuboidal nucleocapsid with two copies of a positive-sense, single-stranded RNA genome. *(bar = 100 nm)*

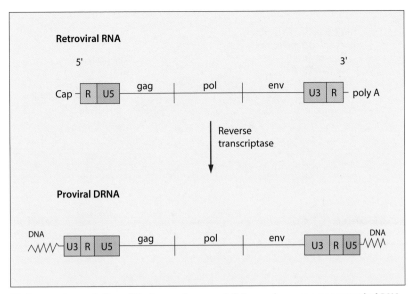

41 Reverse transcription of the human immunodeficiency virus genome to proviral DNA, which is inserted into the chromosome of the host cell.

There are three major subfamilies of the retroviridae. The spumaviruses induce intense vacuolation of the infected cell, resembling foam (Greek, *spuma* = foam). There are no proven disease associations. The lentiviruses have a long incubation period (Latin, *lentus* = slow). The major human pathogens are human immunodeficiency viruses (HIV) 1 and 2, both of which can result in the development of AIDS. HIV-1 attaches to cells bearing its receptor (the CD4 antigen) and penetrates them using glycoprotein spikes on the viral surface (**42**). These spikes are composed of two glycoproteins (gp41 and gp120) encoded by the *env* region of the genome. The capsid and matrix proteins (e.g. p24, p17) are encoded by the *gag* (group-specific antigen) region.

The oncornaviruses are not a definitive subfamily and comprise four distinct morphological subgroups. This is based largely on their electron microscopic appearance on the examination of thin sections of cells (**43**). Type A particles are 60–90 nm in diameter and occur intracellularly. Type B particles are seen following the budding of a preformed capsid through the cell surface. They are 125–130 nm in diameter with an eccentrically sited electron dense core. Murine mammary tumour virus is characteristic of the group. Type C particles have a nucleocapsid that assembles at the plasma membrane at the time of budding, are 80–120 nm in diameter and contain a central electron-dense core. C-type retroviruses include the murine, feline

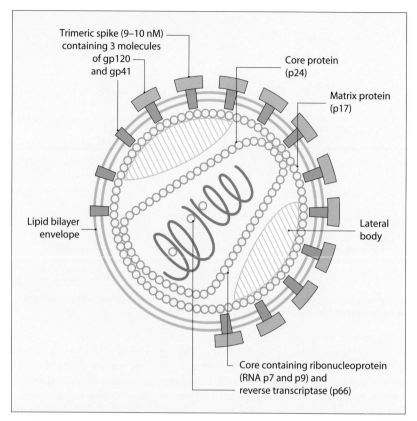

Trimeric spike (9–10 nM)
containing 3 molecules
of gp120
and gp41

Core protein
(p24)

Matrix protein
(p17)

Lipid bilayer
envelope

Lateral
body

Core containing ribonucleoprotein
(RNA p7 and p9) and
reverse transcriptase (p66)

42 Diagram of the structure and polypeptides of human immunodeficiency virus.

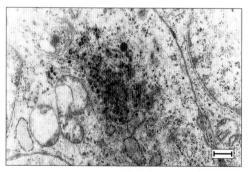

**43 Thin-section electron
micrograph of intracellular
nucleocapsids of B-type
oncornaviruses.** *(bar = 200 nm)*

and simian leukemia viruses. Type D particles have a characteristic bar-shaped core within the envelope, which does not have a surface fringe. Human T-cell leukaemia virus 1 is a C-type virus that causes tropical spastic paresis and adult T-cell leukaemia in man.

■ DNA VIRUSES

The infections caused by DNA viruses are shown in **44**.

Parvoviridae

These are the smallest of the viruses (18–21 nm). They are unenveloped viruses with a single-stranded, linear genome (5 kb) that is mostly negative sense (**45**). Parvovirus B19 is the human pathogen. In children, it causes an acute febrile illness called erythema infectiosum, fifth disease or 'slapped cheek' syndrome. In adults, it may also cause a prolonged arthritis. The virus infects, in particular, erythroid precursor cells in the bone marrow (the P blood group antigen being the receptor). In patients with hemolytic anemia (e.g. hereditary spherocytosis, thalassemia), infection can result in aplastic crises in which the blood hemoglobin level can drop precipitately. Parvovirus may also cross the placenta to infect the fetus, resulting in stillbirth, abortion or hydrops fetalis in 5–7% of cases. Diagnosis is by detection of the genome or of IgM anti-parvovirus.

Papovaviridae

There are two subfamilies in the papovaviridae. The polyomaviruses (JC and BK) rarely cause disease in man. Both are persistently excreted principally in urine following the initial infection. JC virus can cause a severe neurological infection (progressive multifocal leukoencephalopathy) in the immuno-compromised patient. The human papillomaviruses (HPVs) form a large grouping of unenveloped cuboidal DNA viruses (**46**). They have a circular, double-stranded genome (approximately 8 kbp). They are difficult to grow since they require differentiated skin to support replication. They are subdivided into genotypes (of which there are over 100) on the relatedness of DNA sequences. They are responsible for cutaneous (e.g. HPV1) and genital (e.g. HPV12) warts. There is a very strong association between certain HPV types (e.g. HPV16, HPV18, HPV 33) and carcinoma of the cervix.

Adenoviridae

These are eicosahedral, unenveloped viruses (**47**) with a linear, double-stranded DNA genome (36–38 kbp). There are approximately 42 adenovirus serotypes; different serotypes have different disease associations, and, as with enteroviruses, infection can be asymptomatic. Up to 10% of cases of pneumonia in children may be caused by adenovirus types 1, 2, 3, 5 and 7, and some serotypes can also cause a pertussis-like syndrome.

INFECTIONS BY DNA VIRUSES

	Major infections	Less common infections	Vaccine preventable	Incubation period	Period of infectivity
Parvovirus	Erythema infectiosum (fifth disease)	Arthralgia, aplastic crises, hydrops fetalis	No	18–21 days	5 days (in blood 8–14 days post infection)
Papovaviridae					
Polyomavirus (JC, BK)	Asymptomatic	Progressive multifocal leukoencephalopathy (JC)	No	?	Lifetime
Papillomavirus	Warts (cutaneous, mucosal), carcinoma of cervix, anus and rectum	–	No	1–20 months	Until resolution of wart
Hepatitis B	Acute or chronic hepatitis, hepatocellular carcinoma	Asymptomatic (50–60%)	Yes	2–6 months	Can be for life
Adenoviridae	Upper/lower respiratory tract infection (serotypes 1–5, 7, 14, 21) Pneumonia (serotypes 3, 4, 7b, 14, 21) Keratoconjunctivitis (serotypes 18, 19) Pharyngoconjunctival fever (serotypes 3, 7) Diarrheal disease (serotypes 40, 41)	Pertussis (1, 2, 3, 5) Cystitis (1, 4, 7, 11, 21) Asymptomatic (up to 50%)	No	5–10 days	Up to 900 days
Herpesviridae					
HHV-1	'Cold sores', keratitis	Encephalitis	No	3–5 days	Until lesions crust and then for life
HHV-2	Genital herpes	Encephalitis	No	3–5 days	Until lesions crust and then for life
HHV-3	Chickenpox, shingles	Pneumonia, encephalitis	Yes	14–21 days	4 days prior to chickenpox and until lesions crust
HHV-4	Glandular fever	Asymptomatic (80–90%)	No	14–28 days	For life
HHV-5	Upper respiratory tract infection	Asymptomatic (90–95%) pneumonia, congenital disease	No	14–28 days	For life

aSmallpox has been eradicated.

INFECTIONS BY DNA VIRUSES (Cont'd)

	Major infections	Less common infections	Vaccine preventable	Incubation period	Period of infectivity
HHV-6	Exanthem subitum	Asymptomatic (80–90%)	No	5–15 days	For life
HHV-7	Exanthem subitum	Asymptomatic (80–90%)	No	?	?
HHV-8	?	Kaposi's sarcoma	No	?	?
Poxviridae[a]					
Cowpox	Skin lesions		Yes	6–10 days	Until lesion crusts
Monkeypox	Smallpox-like	Encephalitis	Probably	10–14 days	Until lesion crusts
Orf	'Milker's nodes'	Encephalitis	No	3–7 days	Until lesion crusts
Molluscum contagiosum	Skin lesions	–	No	2–7 weeks	Until lesion heals

[a]Smallpox has been eradicated.

44 Infections by DNA viruses. (cont'd)

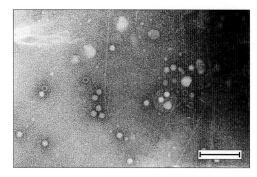

45 Negative-stain electron micrograph of human parvovirus B19. This is an unenveloped, cuboidal virus with a single-stranded DNA genome. It causes 'slapped cheek' syndrome. *(bar = 100 nm)*

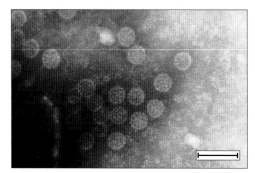

46 Negative-stain electron micrograph of a papillomavirus. This is an unenveloped, cuboidal virus with a circular, double-stranded DNA genome. There are over 60 human papillomavirus genotypes. *(bar = 100 nm)*

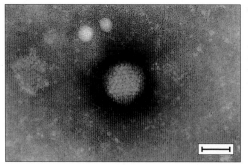

47 Negative-stain electron micrograph of an adenovirus. This is an unenveloped virus with a double-stranded DNA genome. The capsid is made up of 20 triangular facets, each of which is composed of globular capsomers. *(bar = 50 nm)*

Serotypes 40 and 41 cause acute diarrhoeal disease, and types 1–5 have been associated with intussusception. Pharyngoconjunctival fever is caused by serotypes 3 and 7a, and epidemic keratoconjunctivitis by serotypes 3, 4, 7 and 8. Diagnosis is by viral culture, detection of the viral genome by PCR, detection of viral antigen (for Ad40/41) or serology.

Hepadnaviridae

Hepatitis B virus is a small (42 nm), enveloped virus with an eicosahedral nucleocapsid (**48**). Its DNA genome (3.2 kbp) is double stranded, one strand forming a complete loop and the complementary strand a partial loop. HBV is a cause of parenterally acquired hepatitis and has a long (2–6 month) incubation period. In a proportion of patients (especially when infection is neonatally acquired), the infection is not cleared by the immune system but persists in the hepatocytes. Persistent infection may ultimately result in chronic hepatic disease or even hepatocellular carcinoma. Patients with persistent HBV infection may have whole virus particles (Dane particles) and/or tubular and vesicular surface antigen (HBsAg) particles in their bloodstream (**49**). The detection of HBsAg in the blood of a patient without acute hepatitis indicates persistent infection. The detection of HBeAg indicates that these are high-risk carriers who could transmit infection by the transfer of a small volume of blood, for example a needle-stick injury. If the donor is e antigen negative, it is likely that a large amount of blood (e.g. a blood transfusion) would need to be transferred to transmit infection.

Herpesviridae

The herpesviruses are a large family of enveloped viruses with an eicosahedral nucleocapsid (**50**). They have a double-stranded, linear genome (120–200 kbp). There are currently eight human herpesviruses (HHV-1 to HHV-8), and, following initial infection, each becomes established as a latent or persistent infection. Herpes simplex virus type 1 (HHV-1) remains latent

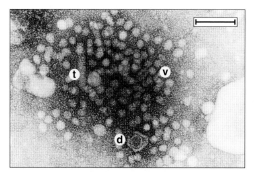

48 Negative-stain electron micrograph of plasma from a patient with acute hepatitis B virus infection. The complete virus (Dane) particles (**d**) have a lipid envelope with a loop of double-stranded DNA genome in a cuboidal nucleocapsid. The tubular (**t**) and vesicular (**v**) particles comprise only viral lipid envelope. *(bar = 100 nm)*

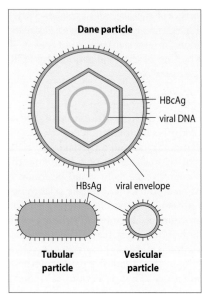

Dane particle

HBcAg
viral DNA

HBsAg   viral envelope

**Tubular
particle**

**Vesicular
particle**

**49 Diagram showing the antigens of
hepatitis B virus.**

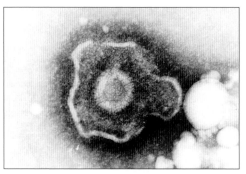

**50 Negative-stain electron
micrograph of herpes simplex
virus.** This is an enveloped virus
with a cuboidal capsid and a linear,
double-stranded DNA genome.
There are eight different human
herpesviruses. *(bar = 100 nm)*

in the trigeminal ganglion and can reactivate and recrudesce to produce cold
sores or keratitis (it is the most common infective cause of blindness in
developed countries). Herpes simplex virus type 2 (HHV-2) causes genital
herpes. Varicella-zoster virus (HHV-3) causes chickenpox and subsequently
reactivates to produce shingles. Epstein–Barr virus (EBV) is also known as
HHV-4 and causes glandular fever. The infection is also known as infectious
mononucleosis since the examination of a peripheral blood film reveals the
presence of large irregular mononuclear cells (**51**). These are T-lymphocytes
that have become activated in an attempt to kill the EBV-infected

B-lymphocytes. Cytomegalovirus (CMV, HHV-5) infection is usually asymptomatic but can cross the placenta to infect the fetus. In such circumstances, it is the most common infective cause of mental retardation. HHV-6, and to a certain extent HHV-7, causes exanthem subitum in young children. The recently described HHV-8 is the cause of Kaposi's sarcoma in both HIV-infected and HIV-uninfected individuals.

Poxviridae
These are the largest (350 × 400 nm) and most complex of the viruses. They can have a lipid envelope (**52**), but this is not an absolute necessity for infectivity. Their capsid symmetry is complex, and they have a double-stranded, linear DNA genome (130–280 kbp). The orthopoxviruses include smallpox (which has been eliminated) monkeypox and cowpox. Of the parapoxviruses, only one, orf, is of importance in human infections (**53**). Molluscum contagiosum is an, as yet, unclassified poxvirus that has not been maintained in artificial culture. On electron microscopy, it has been described as resembling a ball of string (**54**).

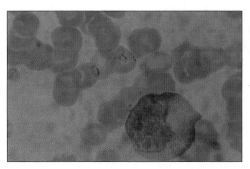

51 Peripheral blood film from a patient with glandular fever (infectious mononucleosis) caused by Epstein–Barr virus (HHV-4). The large, irregular, mononuclear cells are activated T-lymphocytes.

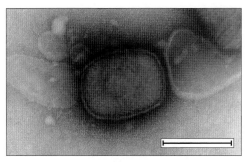

52 Negative-stain electron micrograph of smallpox virus. Although a lipid envelope is visible, this is not necessary for infectivity. *(bar = 300 nm)*

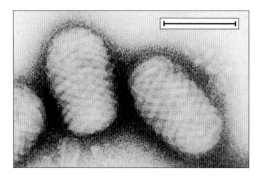

53 Negative-stain electron micrograph of orf, a parapox virus. This complex DNA virus has a double-stranded, linear genome. The regular surface structure is characteristic of parapoxviruses. *(bar = 50 nm)*

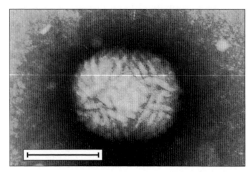

54 Negative-stain electron micrograph of molluscum contagiosium virus. This virus has not been maintained in artificial culture. It is described as resembling a ball of string. *(bar = 300 nm)*

■ DIAGNOSTIC VIROLOGY

Although the presence of a virus infection can on occasion be inferred from non-specific measurements such as presence of lymphocytosis (e.g. in CSF or blood), the precise diagnosis depends upon the detection of virus, viral antigens, viral genome or a serological response to the virus (55).

Detection of Virus
Negative-stain Electron Microscopy
This provides a rapid and specific diagnosis of most viral diarrheas but has also been used to detect respiratory viral infection (56). For viruses to be seen, the sample needs to contain at least 10^6 particles per ml. The sensitivity and specificity can be improved by the addition of specific antisera (immuno-electron microscopy).

Culture
Virus culture can be in whole animals (e.g. suckling mice for coxsackie B viruses), embryonated eggs (e.g. influenza, pox viruses) or cultured cells. Animals are rarely used nowadays for virus isolation.

DIAGNOSTIC METHODS IN VIROLOGY		
Method	**Rapidity of method**	**Sensitivity/specificity**
Detection of virus		
Electron microscopy	Rapid	High
Culture[a]	Moderate (1–7 days)	High
Histology (inclusions)[a]	Moderate (1–14 days)	Low
Detection of viral antigens[a]		
ELISA	Rapid	High
Latex particle agglutination	Rapid	Moderate
Radio-immunoassay	Moderate (1–5 days)	High
Immunofluorescence	Rapid	High
Detection of viral genome		
RNA polyacrylamide gel electrophoresis[b]	Moderate (24–36 h)	High
Genome hybridization	Moderate (1–5 days)	Moderate
Genome amplification by polymerase chain reaction	Moderate (24–72 h)	High
Detection of serological response		
IgM response, e.g. for hepatitis A virus by ELISA	Rapid	High
Rising titre by:		
complement fixation	Slow[c]	High/moderate
hemagglutination inhibition	Slow	High
neutralization	Slow	High
latex particle agglutination	Slow	Moderate
ELISA	Slow	High
radio-immunoassay	Slow	High
immunofluorescence	Slow	High

[a]Not available for all viruses. [b]For rotavirus and picobirnavirus. [c]Requires acute and convalescent sera (at least 2 weeks between).

55 Diagnostic methods in virology.

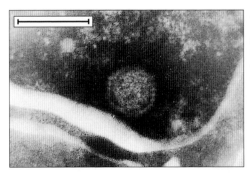

56 Direct negative-stain electron micrograph of bronchial secretions from a child with bronchiolitis obliterans.
Adenovirus was grown from the secretions. *(bar = 200 nm)*

Embryonated chickens' eggs can be used for the isolation of many different viruses. Different viruses require different inoculation sites (**57**). Influenza viruses, for example, are cultured in the amniotic cavity, parainfluenza viruses in the allantoic cavity, St Louis encephalitis virus in the yolk sac and poxviruses on the chorio-allantoic membrane (**58**). Cell lines are, however, available for the culture of most viruses, embryonated eggs being used less and less frequently. In fact, the major use of embryonated eggs is in the large-scale culture of influenza and measles viruses for vaccine production.

The ability to culture human and other mammalian cells has led to great advances in animal virology since they have provided a ready substrate for viral culture. Mammalian cells can be readily grown in plastic flasks containing appropriate growth medium (**59**) either attached to the plastic

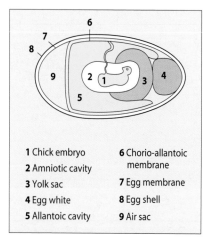

57 Diagram of a fertile hen's egg approximately 10 days old.

1 Chick embryo
2 Amniotic cavity
3 Yolk sac
4 Egg white
5 Allantoic cavity
6 Chorio-allantoic membrane
7 Egg membrane
8 Egg shell
9 Air sac

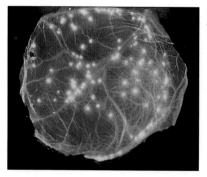

58 Chorio-allantoic membrane showing characteristic poxvirus lesions.

surfaces or in suspension. Cells may be derived directly from living normal tissue, these then being called primary cell cultures. These tend to have a limited lifespan. Transformed cells either derived from malignant tumors or even transformed in vitro provide rapidly growing immortal cell lines. Some cells are fibroblastic (**60**) in appearance (e.g. MRC-5), some resemble epithelial cells (e.g. HEp-2: **61**), and some grow only in suspension and are derived from lymphoblastic (e.g. Raji) or macrophage/monocyte (e.g. U937) precursors. No one cell line will support the growth of all viruses, so viral diagnostic laboratories maintain a range of cell lines.

Following inoculation and growth, viruses can be detected by their cytopathic effect (CPE). The time taken for the CPE to appear varies with different viruses; for example, that of herpes simplex (**62**) takes under 24 h, whereas cytomegaloviruses can take up to 5 days (**63**). For some viruses, the CPE provides a specific diagnosis (e.g. **62**, **63**); for others (e.g. enteroviruses) it is less clear cut (**64**). In some cases, little or no CPE is produced, and virus is detected by other biological activities such as hemadsorption, interference or antigen production. Hemadsorption (**65**) occurs, for example, when the

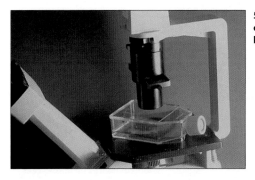

59 Disposable plastic flasks containing monolayers of cells bathed in growth medium.

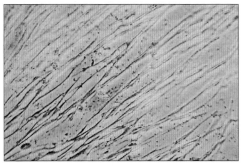

60 Monolayer of human embryo lung fibroblasts (MRC-5). The cells are spindle shaped.

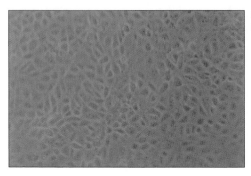

61 Monolayer of African green monkey kidney (Vero) cells.

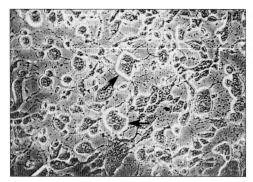

62 Typical cytopathic effect of herpes simplex virus on African green monkey kidney (Vero) cells. The plaques (arrows) consist of fused cells.

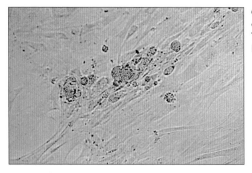

63 Typical cytopathic effect of cytomegalovirus on MRC-5 cells. The large refractile cells are infected by the virus.

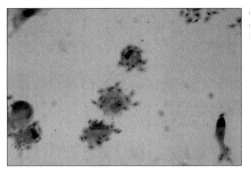

64 Cytopathic effect induced by poliovirus on Vero cells. The cells are killed, but a similar picture can be induced by other viruses and some toxins.

65 Hemadsorption of chicken erythrocytes to influenza virus-infected cells.

hemagglutinin spikes of influenza virus are expressed on the surface of infected cells. When erythrocytes are added, they adhere focally to the infected cell. A variety of immunoassays are used to detect viral growth, either for rapid diagnosis prior to development of the CPE (**66**) or for viruses that do not produce a CPE. In most cases, the confirmation of virus growth and identity can be obtained by negative-stain electron microscopy of the tissue culture fluid.

Inclusions

Finally, it is possible to detect viruses in tissue or even peripheral blood cells either by the presence of inclusions or by the detection of viral antigens. Viral inclusions are aggregates of viral particles (**67**) and can be intranuclear or intracytoplasmic depending upon the site of viral replication and assembly. Rabies virus produces intracytoplasmic inclusions in brain cells called Negri bodies (**68**). Herpesviruses such as varicella-zoster (**69**) and CMV (**70**) produce intranuclear inclusions. Indeed, perinatal infection with CMV is also called cytomegalic inclusion disease. Infected cells are large and show characteristic 'owl's eye' intranuclear inclusions (**70**). Simple histological stains are used to demonstrate such inclusions, but their sensitivity and specificity are not high.

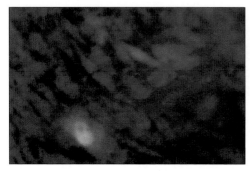

66 The direct early antigen fluorescent focus (DEAFF) assay. The MRC-5 cells infected with cytomegalovirus are stained with fluorescein-conjugated antibody to cytomegalovirus early antigen. This antigen appears within 24–36 h of adding the virus to the cells.

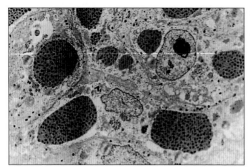

67 Thin-section electron micrograph of cowpox inclusions. They form intracytoplasmic inclusions that can also be stained by Giemsa for light microscopy.

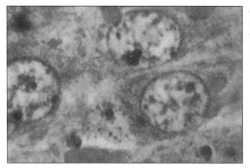

68 The pink cytoplasmic inclusions characteristic of rabies virus infection. They are found in brain cells and are called Negri bodies.

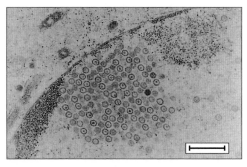

69 Intranuclear inclusions of varicella-zoster virus, which can also be visualized by Giemsa staining and light microscopy. *(bar = 400 nm)*

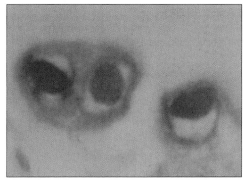

70 Typical 'owl's eye' intranuclear inclusions of cytomegalovirus-infected cells.

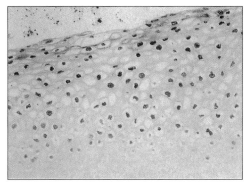

71 Cervical intraepithelial neoplasia grade 1 cells stained with alkaline phosphatase coupled to a monoclonal anti-human papillomavirus (HPV) antibody. The cells expressing HPV antigens are stained blue.

The sensitivity and specificity can be increased by using specific antiviral antisera to stain the inclusions by, for example, immunoperoxidase or immuno-alkaline phosphatase (71).

Detection of Viral Antigens

In these assays, antisera (mono- or polyclonal) are used to detect viral antigen, either free in body fluids or on exfoliated cells or white blood cells. Such assays can be highly sensitive since they can also detect antigens from disrupted virus particles that would not be cultivable or visible by electron microscopy. They are, however, 'pathogen specific'; i.e. a separate immuno-assay must be employed for each pathogen, in contrast to electron microscopy or culture, which are 'catch-all' techniques. The immunoassays vary according to the method used for detecting antigen–antibody binding.

Enzyme-linked Immunosorbent Assay (ELISA)

These are antigen-capture ELISAs (72). Such assays are available for a variety of viral enteropathogens (rotavirus, astrovirus, adenovirus 40/41,

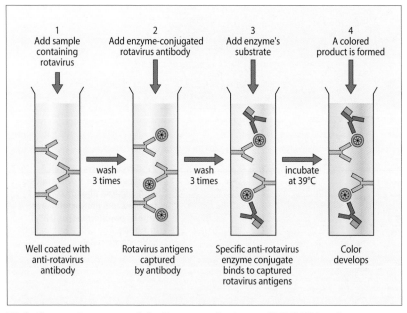

72 Antigen-capture enzyme-linked immunosorbent assay (ELISA). With antigen-capture ELISA, the wells are coated with antibody to the virus. The sample containing virus (**1**) is added, and, after washing several times, enzyme conjugated to an antibody to the virus is added (**2**). Finally, after a further cycle of washing, the enzyme's substrate (**3**) is added. A colored product is formed if the viral antigen is present in the sample (**4**).

Norwalk agent), hepatitis B virus (HBSAg, HBeAg, HBcAg) and HIV (p24). With these, microtitre plate wells are coated with antibody to the specific pathogen. This captures antigen in the biological fluid tested, its presence being detected by adding another antibody to the pathogen with, for example, alkaline phosphatase chemically linked to it. Finally, the enzyme's substrate is added. In each case, a colored product is produced, the intensity of which is proportional to the amount of antigen present (**73**).

Latex particle agglutination
In this system, small latex particles are coated with specific antisera to a particular virus (**74**). If the virus is present in the sample, it cross-links the antibody-coated latex particles, causing the milky latex solution to curdle (**75**). Latex particle agglutination is available for the diagnosis of infection caused by rotavirus or respiratory syncytial virus. In general, the sensitivity and specificity of such assays is less than that of ELISA.

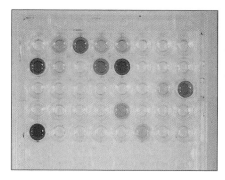

73 Enzyme-linked immunosorbent assay plate showing positive (yellow-brown) and negative wells. In this case, the enzyme used was alkaline phosphatase, and antibody to hepatitis C virus was being detected.

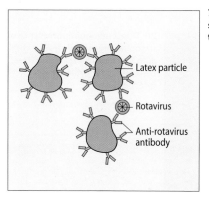

74 Latex particles coated with virus-specific antisera are clumped together by their antigen.

Latex particle

Rotavirus

Anti-rotavirus antibody

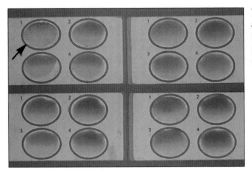

75 Rotavirus latex particle agglutination test. The curdled latex suspensions indicate the presence of rotavirus antigen (arrow).

Immunofluorescence

Immunofluorescence, either direct or indirect, is used to detect viral antigens on or in cells. It provides a rapid and sensitive diagnosis of respiratory tract infection (e.g. respiratory syncytial virus, measles, parainfluenza influenza, measles viruses). These viruses infect cells throughout the respiratory tract. Thus, desquamated cells, which can be obtained by nasopharyngeal aspiration, are fixed on microscope slides and separately stained with fluorescein-tagged specific antibodies to each of the viruses (**76**). The technique is also used for the rapid detection of CMV viremia. CMV p66 antigen can be demonstrated in peripheral blood neutrophils (**77**).

Detection of Viral Genome
RNA Polyacrylamide Gel Electrophoresis (RNA-PAGE)
This is possible only for the direct detection of rotavirus (**29**) or picobirnavirus and is possible only because their genomes are double-stranded RNA and they are excreted in very large quantities in the feces.

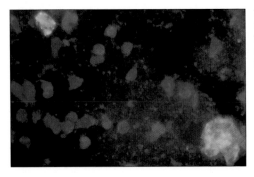

76 Direct immunofluorescence of nasopharyngeal cells from a child with bronchiolitis resulting from respiratory syncytial virus infection.

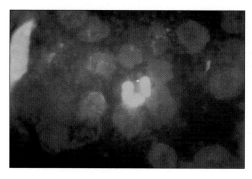

77 Direct immunofluorescence of peripheral blood neutrophils from a patient with acute cytomegalovirus (CMV) infection. Antibody to CMV p66 protein conjugated to fluorescein is used to detect neutrophils containing CMV.

Genome Hybridization

This depends upon the ability of viral DNA or RNA to bind specifically (hybridize) to complementary strains of DNA generated either artificially (usually oligonucleotides) or from cloned virus genome (**78**). The binding is detected by incorporating a radiolabel or an enzyme system into the probe nucleic acid. Radioactive labels are detected using X-ray film, usually as a dot blot. This is the most sensitive detection system but takes several days for the X-ray film to fog and radiolabels are not universally available. Incorporating an enzyme such as peroxidase or alkaline phosphatase (usually via biotinylated nucleotides) allows detection using an ELISA format. Genome hybridization can also be used for the direct detection of virus infection in histological section (**78,79**).

Genome Amplification

With recent developments in molecular biology, it has become possible to amplify fragments of the viral genome in patient's samples. A variety of methods has been developed, including ligase chain reaction and the Q-β system. However, the first method developed and the method most

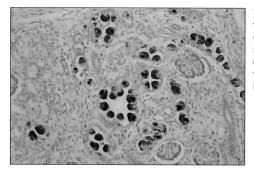

78 Section of kidney from a renal transplant patient with cytomegalovirus infection. The section has been stained with a cytomegalovirus DNA probe linked to alkaline phosphatase. The infected nuclei are stained red.

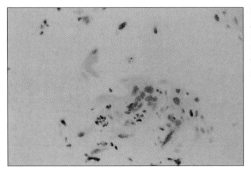

79 Section of esophagus from an AIDS patient with herpes simplex (HSV) esophagitis. The section has been stained with HSV-DNA linked to peroxidase. The infected cells are stained brown.

frequently employed is the PCR. In this, double-stranded DNA is first melted to separate the strands. The sample is mixed with primers that are complementary to sequences of nucleotides (approximately 20) on the two DNA strands. Thus primers are chosen so that they are at either end of a sequence of 50–1000 bases (**80**). As the DNA cools, the excess of primer binds to the complementary sequences on the target DNA, and nucleotides are added sequentially by the thermostable *taq* (from *Theramus aquaticus*) DNA polymerase. This generates two copies of the target DNA. The mixture is reheated to separate the double-stranded DNA and allowed to cool so that the primers can bind and nucleotides be added. The *taq* enzyme is used since it is not denatured by the repeated heating and cooling. After 30–80 cycles of heating and cooling carried out automatically using a thermal cycler (**81**), the amplified DNA can then be detected by electrophoresis on an agarose gel (**82**). It is, however, important to show that the amplified DNA is of the expected target, either by restriction endonuclease digestion (**83**) or by DNA hybridization.

The method can be modified to detect RNA viruses by incorporating a reverse transcriptase step before starting PCR. Theoretically, just one copy of the viral genome can be detected in a sample, but in practice, larger amounts are needed. The sample may also contain inhibitors of the reaction that may cause false-negative results. The method is exquisitely sensitive, and false positives can occur from contamination of the sample by exogenous target. It is thus advisable to have well-separated areas for preparation of samples, thermal cycling and detection of amplified product. The sensitivity and specificity of PCR can be improved by using 'nested' primers (**84**). These tests have now become automated (**85**), and detection systems for a number of viruses are commercially available. It is now even possible to estimate viral load using, for example, light-cycler technology (**86,87**). Measurement of viral load, for example in HIV infection, is needed to monitor treatment and assess prognosis.

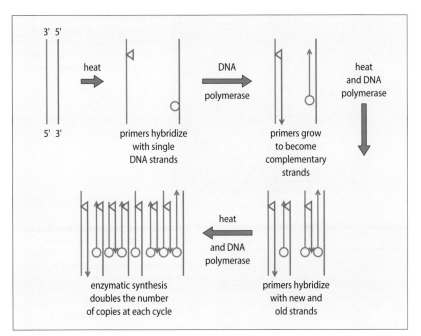

80 Polymerase chain reaction.

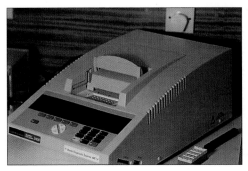

81 Thermal cycler used in the polymerase chain reaction.

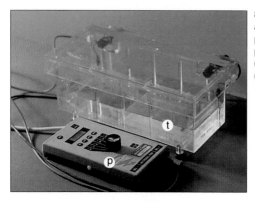

82 Equipment needed for agarose gel electrophoresis of polymerase chain reaction products, including a power pack (p) and an electrophoresis tank (t).

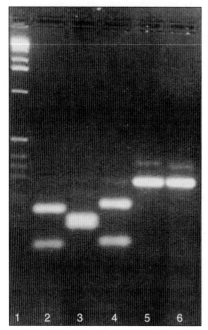

83 Ethidium bromide-stained agarose gels of restriction endonuclease-digested reverse transcriptase–polymerase chain reaction products amplified from the NP protein gene of respiratory syncytial virus. Lane 1 contains a 'lambda-ladder' of molecular weight markers. Lanes 2 and 4, lanes 5 and 6, and lane 3 show three separate NP types respectively.

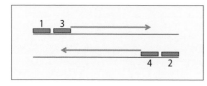

84 Nested primers increase the sensitivity and specificity of the polymerase chain reaction.

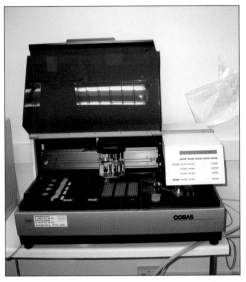

85 Example of an automated polymerase chain reaction machine.

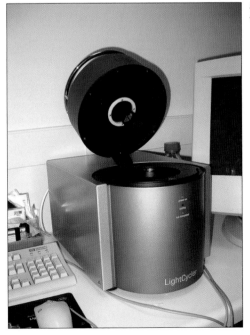

86 Light cycler for measuring viral load.

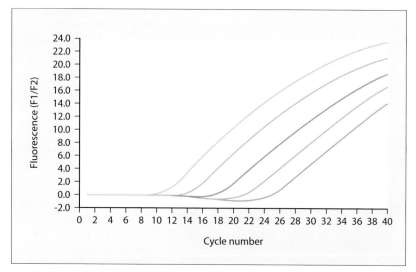

87 Print-out from a light cycler showing increasing signal with number of cycles.

Detection of Serological Response

Following initial challenge with an antigen (such as a viral or bacterial pathogen), a primary antibody response is mounted (88). This takes approximately 2 weeks to reach maximum level, and the antibody produced is principally of the IgM class. On subsequent challenge, a secondary response is elicited that is much more rapid (of the order of 24–48 h) and produces a higher level of high-affinity antibody, principally of the IgG class (88). This, of course, is the aim of immunization. However, from the above, it follows that the serological diagnosis of viral infection will most often not provide an answer until the patient has recovered. Acute (taken on presentation) and convalescent (taken 10–14 days later) serum samples are required and, in general, a four-fold rise in titre is taken to indicate infection.

IgM Detection

IgM is the first class of antibody to be produced, and its detection can provide earlier evidence of infection. It is used, for example, in the early diagnosis of EBV or *Mycoplasma pneumoniae* infections. They are, however, usually negative until the fifth or sixth day of illness. The detection of IgM to hepatitis A virus provides a rapid diagnosis (89) since this antibody appears at the time the patient becomes jaundiced.

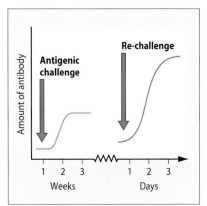

88 Primary and secondary immune responses. On first exposure to an antigen (vaccine or pathogen), peak antibody production takes 2–3 weeks, the antibody produced being primarily of IgM and low affinity. On second exposure, the peak response is higher and more rapid (2–3 days). The antibody produced is of much higher affinity and is predominantly IgG and IgA.

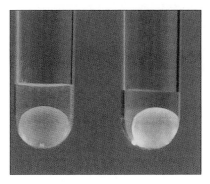

89 Detection of hepatitis A virus (HAV) IgM. The bead is coated with anti-IgM. It is placed in the patient's serum, where it traps IgM. The bead is then placed in a solution containing enzyme-linked HAV antigen. If the patient has HAV IgM, the bead will trap the antigen–enzyme complex. Finally, the complex is placed in a solution of the appropriate substrate. A positive result is seen by the development of a colored product.

Detection of Rising Titre

A variety of techniques is available to detect specific antiviral antibodies. Complement fixation (**90**) is a tried and tested method but suffers from somewhat lower sensitivity, is technically challenging and of course detects IgG and IgM antibodies combined. It is less and less used as a diagnostic tool but can still be of value (**91**).

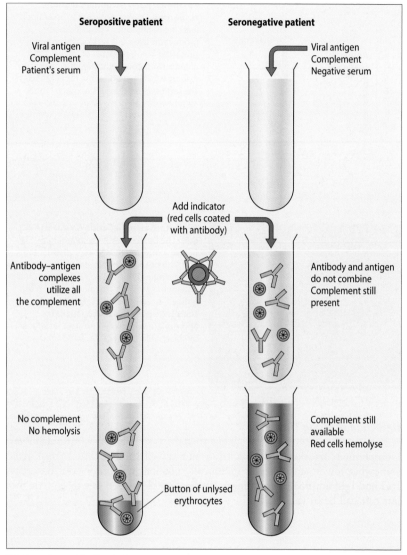

90 Complement fixation test.

Antibodies to influenza, mumps and parainfluenza viruses can bind to their respective haemagglutinin spikes and prevent the viruses binding to their receptors (sialic acid) on erythrocytes. Levels of antibody to these viruses can thus be estimated by hemagglutination inhibition (**92**). For estimation of neutralizing antibodies, their ability to prevent viral replication is measured. Not all antibodies produced in response to infection are neutralizing, and the technique is primarily used for virus typing (e.g. differentiating ECHO viruses). ELISA is perhaps the most versatile and sensitive of the techniques. Two formats are available (**93**). In the first, viral antigen is coated on to the wells, to which dilutions of the sera are added. To detect binding of the patient's serum to the antigen, anti-human antibody coupled to an appropriate enzyme is added. By using anti-human IgG–, IgA–, IgM– or even IgE– enzyme conjugates, the different classes of antiviral antibody can be detected. In the second format, the wells are coated with anti-human IgA, IgM or IgG, which captures all the antibody of that class in the

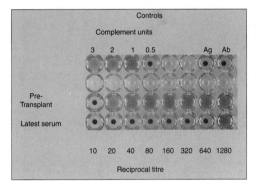

91 World Health Organization tray showing the complement fixation test. Hemolysis means there is no antiviral antibody; a lack of hemolysis indicates that antiviral antibody is present. The serum taken from the patient pre-transplant shows anti-cytomegalovirus at a dilution of 1:10. The sample, taken 8 weeks post-transplantation, during a rejection episode, shows that the antibody titre has risen to 1:640.

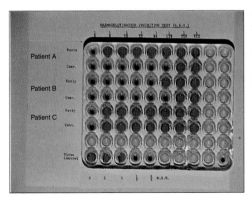

92 Hemagglutination inhibition test. A button of cells in the well indicates that the erythrocytes have not been agglutinated by influenza virus because specific antibody is present. Patient A shows an hemagglutination inhibition titre of 1:4 during the early part of his illness, but 3 weeks later the titre has risen to 1:128.

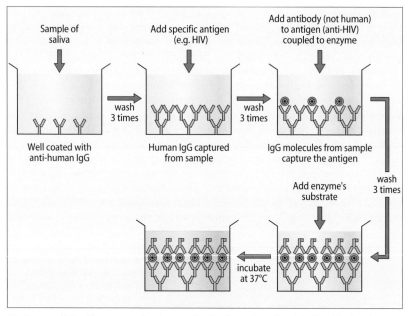

93 Enzyme-linked immunosorbent assay for the detection of antiviral antibody. The antibody-capture format provides a more sensitive assay for IgG, IgM or IgA in saliva.

sample. The specific viral antigen is then added, followed by an enzyme–antibody conjugate against the viral antigen. This method is most useful when the antibody level is relatively low, for example for detecting specific IgA, IgM or IgG in saliva.

Chapter 4

BACTERIA AND DISEASE

Infections caused by bacteria are responsible for diseases ranging from a mild tonsillitis to epidemics of cholera and plague. Bacteria are remarkably adaptable microorganisms. They may cause severe disease or innocently colonize the skin. They may survive and multiply in the environment, and they may form spores that can survive for decades. Some bacteria are primarily parasites of animals, only infecting humans as a chance event, whereas others can survive only by intimate contact with their human host. Whereas most bacteria replicate in hours or days, some are much slower growers, leading to chronic infections and difficulties in treatment. As well as diversity in their ecology, bacteria have the potential for variation in their genetic composition. Many bacteria contain plasmid DNA, which enables the transfer of genetic material both within and between species. This genetic adaptability can enhance both pathogenic mechanisms and resistance to antimicrobial agents.

■ BACTERIAL STRUCTURE

Bacteria are prokaryotes. Their DNA is not in a nucleus but free in the cytoplasm, and they have no internal organelles (**94**). Many bacteria contain extrachromosomal DNA supercoiled loops termed plasmids. Within the cytoplasm, there are no organelles other than ribosomes, which are smaller in size than those of eukaryotic cells. Bacteria other than *Mycoplasma* are surrounded by a complex cell wall, which differs between Gram-positive and Gram-negative bacteria. Many bacteria have external appendages such as flagella, pili, curli or capsules.

Both Gram-positive and Gram-negative bacteria have a plasma membrane formed by a lipid bilayer together with integral membrane proteins, and in both the principal structural component of the cell wall is a three-dimensional framework of a heteropolymer of N-acetylglucosamine and N-acetylmuramic acid, and five amino acids termed peptidoglycan.

In Gram-positive bacteria, the cell wall consists almost exclusively of this peptidoglycan layer with attached teichoic acid polymers (**95**). Gram-negative bacteria have a more complex cell wall. The peptidoglycan layer is thinner than in Gram-positive organisms and is surrounded by an outer

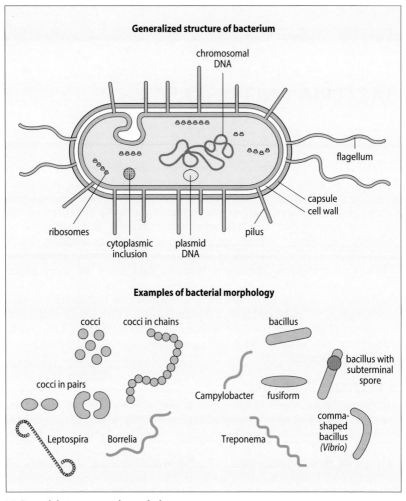

Generalized structure of bacterium

chromosomal
DNA

flagellum

capsule
cell wall

ribosomes

cytoplasmic
inclusion

plasmid
DNA

pilus

Examples of bacterial morphology

cocci

cocci in chains

bacillus

bacillus with
subterminal
spore

cocci in pairs

Campylobacter

fusiform

comma-
shaped
bacillus
(Vibrio)

Leptospira

Borrelia

Treponema

94 Bacterial structure and morphology.

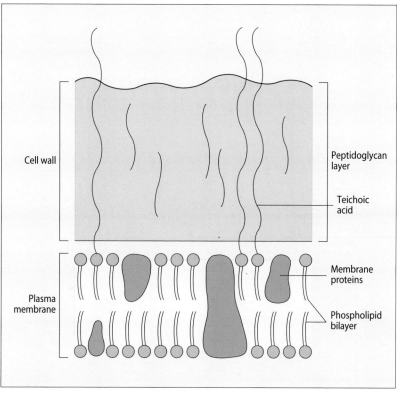

95 Cell wall structure of a Gram-positive bacterium.

membrane comprising phospholipids, lipopolysaccharides, ergosterol and lipoproteins (**96**). This lipopolysaccharide component of the Gram-negative cell wall is amphipathic, with a hydrophilic polysaccharide region external to the cell which imparts O- or somatic antigenicity, and a hydrophobic region, lipid A, embedded in the lipid bilayer. Lipid A is endotoxin, which contributes to Gram-negative bacterial pathogenicity.

■ BACTERIAL CLASSIFICATION AND CULTURE

The shape of bacteria, and their staining properties, form the basis for classification. Bacteria may be spherical (cocci), rod shaped (bacilli) or intermediate (cocco-bacilli). Most bacteria can be stained by the Gram reaction, Gram-positive bacteria being blue-purple and Gram-negative bacteria pink. Mycobacteria (eg. *M. tuberculosis*) are stained by the Ziehl–Neelsen

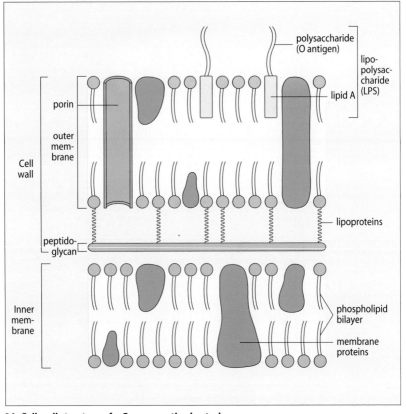

96 Cell wall structure of a Gram-negative bacterium.

technique, the stained bacteria being pink. **97–100** show the classification of the medically important bacteria, many of which are illustrated in the following sections.

Most bacteria can be grown on artificial culture media, which provide the necessary nutrients for growth. Some bacteria are obligate intracellular parasites; these are *Rickettsia*, *Chlamydia* and *Coxiella* spp and can be cultivated only in vivo or in cell culture systems.

Bacteria that can be cultivated may be grown on non-selective culture media, such as nutrient agar or blood agar, which allow a wide range of bacteria to grow, or selective media which, because of the selective agents incorporated (e.g. bile in MacConkey media) or antibiotics (e.g. vancomycin, colistin), allow only certain bacteria to grow. Some bacteria are obligate

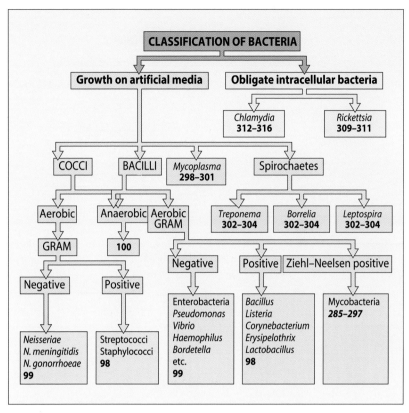

97 Classification of bacteria.

anaerobes and will grow only in an atmosphere devoid of oxygen. In the diagnostic laboratory, different media and culture conditions are used to isolate particular bacteria from clinical specimens (**101**).

Whereas some bacteria may be presumptively identified by characteristic microscopy and culture appearances (e.g. *Vibrio cholerae, Neisseria meningitidis*), further tests are usually necessary to confirm identity. Many of these tests are biochemical, in which bacteria with similar Gram and cultural appearances can be distinguished by carbohydrate fermentation or other biochemical tests (**102**). For some bacteria (e.g. *Salmonella* spp, *N. meningitidis*), subtypes may be distinguished by antigenic differences, determined by agglutination with specific antisera (**103**).

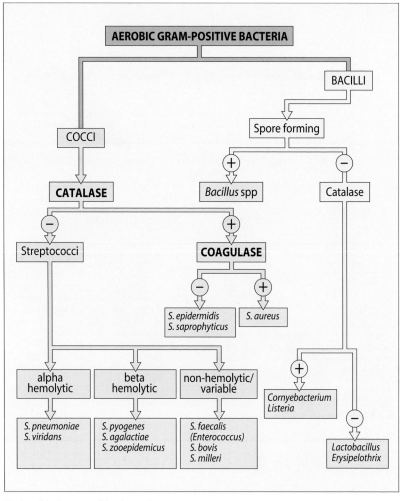

98 Aerobic Gram-positive bacteria.

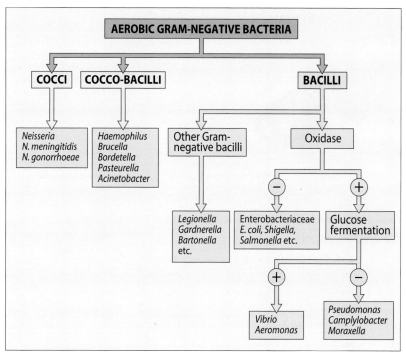

99 Aerobic Gram-negative bacteria.

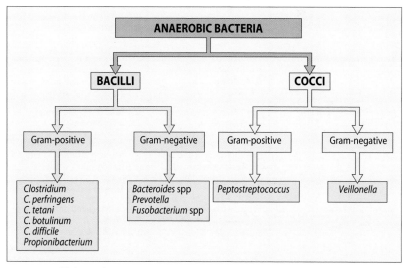

100 Anaerobic bacteria.

BACTERIAL CULTURE MEDIA

Medium	Major ingredients	Uses
Blood agar	Nutrient agar + 5% horse or sheep blood	Non-selective medium for a wide range of non-fastidious Gram-negative and Gram-positive bacteria
Buffered charcoal yeast extract (BCYE) agar	Yeast extract, charcoal, HCl, α-ketoglutarate	Selective for *Legionella* spp
Campylobacter medium	Nutrient agar base with vancomycin, trimethoprim and amphotericin	Selective medium for *Campylobacter* spp
Cefsoludin, irgasan, novobiocin (CIN) agar	Peptone base with antibiotic supplements	Selective medium for *Yersinia* spp
Charcoal cephalexin blood (CCBA) agar	Charcoal agar, sheep blood, cephalexin	Selective medium for *Bordetella* spp
Chocolate (heated blood) agar	Heated blood agar. The cells are lysed and specific growth factors released	Cultivation of *Haemophilus* and *Neisseria* spp
Cycloserine, cefoxitin, fructose agar (CCFA)	Egg yolk base with fructose antibiotics	Selective medium for *Clostridium difficile*
Cystine, lactose, electrolyte-deficient (CLED) agar	Peptone base with lactose and L-cystine. Bromothymol blue indicator inhibits swarming of *Proteus* spp	Isolation of bacteria in urine
Deoxycholate citrate agar	Peptone agar base including lactose, deoxycholate and indicator neutral red	Selective medium for *Salmonella* and *Shigella*
Kanamycin blood agar	Blood agar base with kanamycin	Selective isolation of *Bacteroides* spp
Kligler iron agar (KIA)	Peptone agar base with lactose, glucose, phenol red and ferric citrate	A differential slope medium to distinguish *Shigella* and *Salmonella* and other Enterobacteriaceae
Löwenstein–Jensen (LJ) medium	Egg-based medium with malachite green	Selective medium for mycobacteria
MacConkey agar	Peptone base containing bile salts, lactose and neutral red. Lactose fermenters produce acid and thus pink colonies	A low selectivity medium for enteric bacteria that distinguishes lactose fermenters and non-lactose fermenters
Mannitol salt agar	Peptone base containing mannitol, sodium chloride and phenol red	Selective and differential medium for isolating *Staphylococcus aureus*

101 Bacterial culture media.

BACTERIAL CULTURE MEDIA (Cont'd)		
Medium	**Major ingredients**	**Uses**
Modified New York City (MNYC) medium	Peptone base with yeast and hemoglobin, and antibiotics including vancomycin and colistin	A selective medium to isolate *N. gonorrhoeae* from urogenital specimens
Salmonella–Shigella (SS) agar	Peptone-based medium containing bile salts, lactose, neutral red and ferric citrate	A selective medium to isolate *Salmonella* and *Shigella* spp
Sorbitol MacConkey agar	Peptone base containing bile salts, sorbitol and neutral red	Differentiation of non-sorbitol-fermenting *Escherichia coli* (*E. coli* O157)
Tellurite blood agar	Blood agar with potassium tellurite	Selective medium for *C. diphtheriae*, which reduces tellurite to form black colonies
Thayer–Martin agar	Blood agar base with supplements and antibiotics including colistin and vancomycin	Selective isolation of *Neisseria* spp
Thiosulfate, citrate, bile salt (TCBS) agar	Peptone base including thiosulfate, citrate, sucrose and thymol blue	Selective medium for *Vibrio* spp. *Vibrio cholerae* ferments sucrose and produces yellow colonies
Xylose, lysine, deoxycholate (XLD) agar	Yeast extract with lysine, xylose, lactose and ferric citrate	Selective and differential medium for *Shigella* (pink colonies) and *Salmonella* (pink-black colonies)

101 Bacterial culture media (Cont'd).

■ **AEROBIC GRAM-POSITIVE BACTERIA**

Gram-positive Cocci

The characteristics of Gram-positive cocci are summarized in **104–106** and **116–118**.

Staphylococci

Staphylococci are a major component of the human normal flora but also include species that are important pathogens. On staining, they appear as Gram-positive cocci in clusters (**107–109**). **110** and **111** show the culture appearance of *Staphylococcus epidermidis* and *S. aureus* on blood agar.

BIOCHEMICAL TESTS FOR BACTERIAL IDENTIFICATION

Test	Test principle	Examples of use
Bile solubility	Bile salts dissolve *Streptococcus pneumoniae*	To distinguish *S. pneumoniae* from other alpha hemolytic streptococci
Catalase	Catalase breaks down H_2O_2 to produce bubbles of oxygen	To differentiate streptococci (negative) from staphylococci (positive)
Coagulase	Enzyme coagulase clots plasma	To differentiate coagulase-positive (*Staphylococcus aureus*) and negative staphylococci
Cooked meat medium	Saccharolytic reaction causes reddening of the meat. Proteolytic reaction causes blackening	Distinguishes *Clostridium perfringens* (saccharolytic) from other clostridia
DNAase	Enzyme deoxyribonuclease hydrolyses DNA. Unhydrolysed DNA forms a precipitate with HCl	To distinguish *S. aureus* (positive) from other staphylococci
Dye inhibition test	Growth of different *Brucella* spp is inhibited by the dyes basic fuchsin and thionin	To differentiate *Brucella* spp
Hiss' serum sugars	Detection of growth and acid production from different carbohydrate substrates	To differentiate *Corynebacterium* spp
Indole test	Tryptophan is broken down, with the release of indole, which produces a red color with Kovac's reagent	To distinguish *Escherichia coli* from other Enterobacteriaceae
Koser's citrate test	Growth in citrate medium produces alkaline conditions and the indicator changes from green to blue	To differentiate bacteria that can use citrate as a sole carbon source
Lactose egg yolk medium	Detects lecithinase activity, lactose fermentation, lipase hydrolysis and proteinase activity	Differentiation of *Clostridium* spp
Litmus milk decolorization	Enzymatic reduction and decolorization of litmus milk	Identification of enterococci (positive) and some clostridia

102 Biochemical tests for bacterial identification.

BIOCHEMICAL TESTS FOR BACTERIAL IDENTIFICATION (*Cont'd*)		
Test	**Test principle**	**Examples of use**
Methyl red test	Production of acid in glucose fermentation sufficient to give a red color with the indicator methyl red	Distinguishes *E. coli* and *Enterobacter* spp
Nagler reaction	Detects production of lecithinase and opacity in egg yolk agar	Distinguishes *C. perfringens* from other clostridia
Neisseria carbohydrate fermentation tests	Detects fermentation of glucose, maltose and lactose in *Neisseria* spp	Differentiates *Neisseria gonorrhoeae* (glucose only) from *N. meningitidis* (glucose and maltose) from other *Neisseria*
Nitrate reduction test	The enzyme nitrate reductase reduces nitrate to nitrite	Differentiates nitrate-positive Enterobacteriaceae from other Gram-negative bacteria
Oxidase test	Oxidase enzymes oxidize phenylenediamine, producing a blue color	Assists in the identification of oxidase-positive bacteria, e.g. vibrios, *Neisseriae*
Oxidation-fermentation test	Organisms are incubated in a medium containing glucose (to test for oxidation) and anaerobic (to test for fermentation) conditions	Distinguishes organisms that oxidize glucose (e.g. *Pseudomonas*) from fermenters (e.g. Enterobacteriaceae)
Peptone-water sugars	Series of peptone-waters containing different carbohydrates as substrates	To distinguish different members of the Enterobacteriaceae
Phenylalanine deaminase	Phenylalanine broken down to produce phenylpyruvic acid, which produces a green color with ferric chloride	Differentiates *Proteus* (positive) from other Enterobacteriaceae
Urease test	Urease-producing bacteria hydrolyse urea, producing ammonia, which changes the indicator phenol red to a red color	Differentiates *Proteus* (positive) from other Enterobacteriaceae
Voges–Proskauer (VP) test	Some bacteria ferment glucose with the production of acetoin, which is detected by producing a pink color with creatinine	Distinguishes VP-positive, e.g. *K. pneumoniae* from VP-negative, e.g. *E. coli*, Enterobacteria
X and V test	Some bacteria will only grow in the presence of porphyrin (factor X) and/or NAD (factor V)	Differentiation of *Haemophilus* spp

102 Biochemical tests for bacterial identification (*Cont'd*).

EXAMPLES OF BACTERIAL SUBTYPING BASED ON ANTIGENIC PROPERTIES

Bacteria	Typing system	Antigens detected
Beta hemolytic streptococci	Lancefield grouping	Group-specific cell well carbohydrates; groups A, B, C, D and G most commonly found in human infections
Group A beta hemolytic streptococci	Griffith's typing	Cell wall M proteins differentiate group A streptococci and determine virulence
Streptococcus pneumoniae	Serotyping	Capsular polysaccharides distinguish over 80 serotypes
Neisseria meningitidis	Serogroups	Capsular polysaccharides distinguish 13 serogroups, the major human pathogens being A, B, C and W135
N. meningitidis	Subtypes	Class 2 and 3 outer membrane proteins, e.g. serogroup B, type 15
N. meningitidis	Serotypes (Frasch typing)	Class 1 outer membrane proteins give further differentiation particularly in group B
H. influenzae	Pittman types	Capsular polysaccharides distinguish six types: a–f. Type b responsible for most invasive infections
Salmonella spp	Kaufman–White scheme	Classification of salmonellae based on O (somatic) and H (flagellar) antigens
Shigella spp	Serogroups and serotypes	O antigens define the four major groups: A, *S. dysenteriae*; B, *S. flexneri*; C, *S. boydii*; and D, *S. sonnei*. Also serotypes within groups A, B and C
V. cholerae	Serogrouping	Somatic (O) antigens. Serogroups 01 and 0139 cause cholera
V. cholerae 01	Subtyping	01 antigens A, B and C distinguish Ogawa, Inaba and Hikojima subtypes

103 Examples of bacterial subtyping based on antigenic properties.

GRAM-POSITIVE COCCI INFECTIONS					
Organism	Major infection	Less common infection	Vaccine preventable?	Incubation period	Period of infectivity
Staphylococci					
S. epidermidis	Bacteremia in immuno-compromised	Most commonly associated with indwelling devices	No	–	–
S. saprophyticus	Urinary tract infections		No	–	–
S. aureus	Boils, impetigo, wound infections, osteomyelitis, septicemia	Pneumonia, endocarditis, toxic shock syndrome, food poisoning	No	–	–
Micrococci	Occasional contaminant of clinical specimens				
Streptococci **(a) Beta hemolytic**					
S. pyogenes (group A)	Tonsillitis, impetigo, cellulitis, scarlet fever (rheumatic fever, glomerulo-nephritis)	Puerperal sepsis, erysipelas, septicemia	No	1–3 days	–
S. agalactiae (group B)	Neonatal sepsis	Puerperal sepsis, osteomyelitis	No	–	–
S. zooepidemicus (group C)	Bacteremia		No	–	–

104 Gram-positive cocci. Infections.

The coagulase test is used to distinguish *S. aureus* (coagulase positive) from the other staphylococci (**112**). Staphylococci can also be distinguished by testing for DNAase production. *Staphylococcus aureus* is DNAase positive (**113**). Selective media such as mannitol salt agar may be used for culturing *S. aureus* when screening cases for carriage in epidemiological studies (**114**).

115 shows a culture of micrococcus on blood agar. They are Gram-positive cocci that are rarely of clinical significance.

GRAM-POSITIVE COCCI
SOURCES AND TRANSMISSION OF BACTERIA

Organism	Reservoir			Transmission				Comments
	Man	Animal	Env.	Feco-oral	Droplet	Direct	Nosocomial	
Staphylococcus epidermidis	+	–	–	–	–	+	+	
S. saprophyticus	+	–	–	–	–	+	–	
S. aureus	+	+	+/–	+	+	+	+	Methicillin-resistant strains are an important hospital problem
Micrococci	+	–	+	–	–	+	+/–	
Streptococcus pyogenes	+	–	–	–	+	+	+	
S. agalactiae	+	–	–	–	+	+	–	
S. zooepidemicus	+	+		+	+/–	–	–	Outbreaks have occurred from unpasteurized milk

105 Gram-positive cocci. Sources and transmission of bacteria.

GRAM-POSITIVE COCCI
IDENTIFYING CHARACTERISTICS

Organism	Gram	Culture on blood agar	Biochemical	Other tests
Staphylococcus epidermidis	+ve cocci	Pale colonies	Catalase +ve	Coagulase –ve, mannitol +ve
S. saprophyticus	+ve cocci	Pale colonies	Catalase +ve	Coagulase –ve, mannitol +ve
S. aureus	+ve cocci	Yellow colonies	Catalase +ve	Coagulase +ve
Micrococci	+ve cocci	Yellow-orange colonies	Catalase +ve	coagulase –ve, bacitracin sensitive
Streptococcus pyogenes	+ve cocci in chains	Beta hemolytic	Catalase –ve	Bacitracin sensitive
S. agalactiae	+ve cocci	Beta hemolytic	Catalase –ve	CAMP +ve
S. zooepidemicus	+ve cocci	Beta hemolytic	Catalase –ve	Lancefield group C

106 Gram-positive cocci. Identifying characteristics.

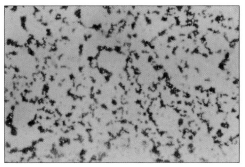

107 *Staphylococcus aureus.* Gram stain showing the typical Gram-positive cocci in clusters. *Staphylococcus aureus* is an important pathogen, causing skin infections, osteomyelitis, septicemia and pneumonia. It is coagulase positive.
(Gram stain, ×1000)

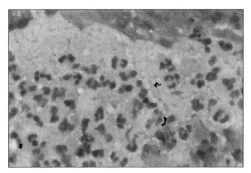

108 *Staphylococcus aureus.* Gram stain of blood culture from a patient with septicemia caused by *S. aureus*. Staphylococcal septicemia may result from the infection of a minor injury.
(Gram stain, ×1000)

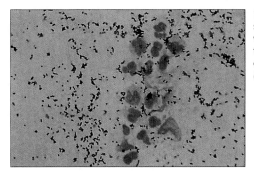

109 *Staphylococcus aureus.* Gram stain of pus from patient with a wound infected with *S. aureus*. Note the Gram-positive cocci and pink-colored pus cells.
(Gram stain, ×1000)

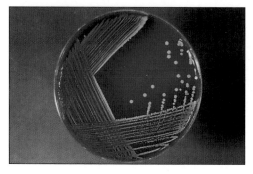

110 *Staphylococcus epidermidis*.
Culture on blood agar showing white colonies. *Staphylococcus epidermidis* is one of the coagulase-negative staphylococci. They are part of the normal skin flora, but may cause infection in neonates, the immunocompromised and patients with indwelling devices. *(Blood agar, 18 h at 37°C)*

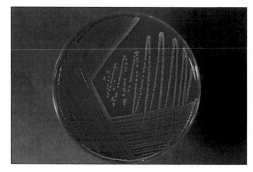

111 *Staphylococcus aureus*.
Culture on blood agar. *Staphylococcus aureus* typically forms yellow or golden colonies, in contrast to the pale colonies of *S. epidermidis* and other coagulase-negative staphylococci. *(Blood agar, 18 h at 37°C)*

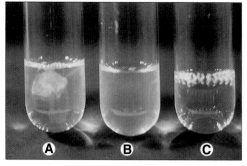

112 Tube coagulase test.
Staphylococcus aureus produces coagulase, which clots plasma. A few drops of a broth culture of the test organism are added to 1:10 diluted plasma in saline and incubated for 2 h at 37°C.
(A) Coagulase-positive *S. aureus*, **(B)** coagulase-negative *S. epidermidis*. A negative control tube is included **(C)**. *(2 h at 37°C)*

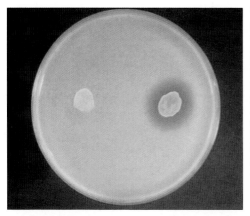

113 DNAase test. Coagulase-positive and negative staphylococci can be distinguished by testing for DNAase production. After overnight incubation on a medium containing DNA, the plate is flooded with weak hydrochloric acid. The acid precipitates unhydrolysed DNA. DNAase-producing colonies are surrounded by clear areas where the DNA has been hydrolysed. *Staphylococcus aureus* is DNAase producing. *(DNAase agar, 18 h at 37°C)*

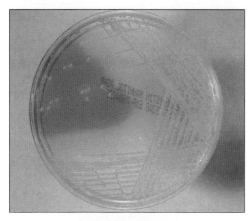

114 *Staphylococcus aureus*. Culture on mannitol salt agar, showing yellow colonies. This is a selective medium for recovering *S. aureus* when screening for carriage in infection control investigations. *(Mannitol salt agar, 18 h at 37°C)*

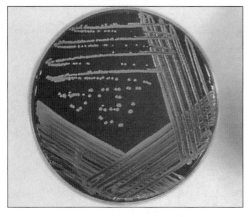

115 Micrococcus. Culture on blood agar, showing pale yellow colonies. Micrococci may occur as contaminants of clinical specimens. *(Blood agar, 18 h at 37°C)*

GRAM-POSITIVE COCCI INFECTIONS					
Organism	Major infection	Less common infection	Vaccine preventable?	Incubation period	Period of infectivity
Streptococci (Cont. from **104**) *(b) Alpha hemolytic*					
S. pneumoniae	Pneumonia, otitis media	Meningitis, septicemia	Yes (some serotypes)	–	–
S. viridans	Dental caries	Subacute bacterial endocarditis	No	–	–
(c) Group D streptococci S. faecalis (enterococci) (*Enterococcus faecalis*)	Urinary tract infections, wound infections, intra-abdominal abscess	Bacteremia, endocarditis	No	–	–
S. bovis	Endocarditis, bacteremia		No	–	–
Other streptococci S. milleri	Intra-abdominal sepsis, wound infections, brain abscess	–	No	–	–

116 Gram-positive cocci. Infections (cont. from **104**).

GRAM-POSITIVE COCCI SOURCES AND TRANSMISSION OF BACTERIA								
	Reservoir			Transmission				
Organism	Man	Animal	Env.	Feco-oral	Droplet	Direct	Nosocomial	Comments
Streptococcus pneumoniae	+	–	–	–	+	–	–	Penicillin-resistant strains increasing
S. viridans	+	–	–	–	+/–	+	–	
Enterococcus faecalis	+	–	–	–	–	+	+	Occasional vancomycin-resistant strains
S. bovis	+	+	–	–	–	+	–	
S. milleri	+	–	–	–	–	+	+	

117 Gram-positive cocci. Sources and transmission of bacteria.

GRAM-POSITIVE COCCI IDENTIFYING CHARACTERISTICS			
Organism	**Gram**	**Culture on blood agar**	**Biochemical and other tests**
Streptococcus pneumoniae	+ve cocci in pairs	Alpha hemolytic 'draughtsman colonies'	Optochin sensitive, +ve bile solubility
S. viridans	+ve cocci	Alpha hemolytic	Optochin resistant, –ve bile solubility
Enterococcus faecalis	+ve cocci	Variable hemolysis	Grows on MacConkey medium, +ve litmus milk test
S. bovis	+ve cocci	Variable hemolysis	No growth in 6.5% NaCl medium
S. milleri	+ve cocci	Small, beta hemolytic colonies	Voges–Proskauer test positive

118 Gram-positive cocci. Identifying characteristics.

Streptococci

Streptococci are Gram-positive cocci that can be distinguished from staphylococci by the catalase test (**119**). *Streptococcus pyogenes*, a pathogen responsible for a range of superficial and deep infections, is seen as chains of cocci in Gram-stained preparations (**120**). **121** shows a Gram stain of *S. agalactiae* (group B *Streptococcus*) from a blood culture of a neonate with septicemia.

Streptococci may be classified according to their hemolysis when cultured on blood agar. **122** shows beta (clear) hemolysis produced by *S. pyogenes*. Beta hemolytic streptococci are divided into Lancefield groups, depending on cell wall polysaccharide antigens (**123**). *Streptococcus pyogenes* is Lancefield group A and *S. agalactiae* Lancefield group B. Alpha hemolysis is a partial hemolysis producing a greenish zone around the colonies. *Streptococcus pneumoniae* (**124**) and *S. viridans* (**125**) show alpha hemolysis. These plates contain optochin discs, which distinguish *S. pneumoniae* (optochin sensitive) from other alpha hemolytic streptococci. *Streptococcus pneumoniae* may be also be distinguished by the bile solubility test (**126**). *Streptococcus pneumoniae* shows characteristic diplococci on Gram staining (**127, 128**).

Streptococci that grow in the intestine are now termed enterococci. They are able to grow on MacConkey medium that contains bile (**129**). Enterococci can be distinguished from other streptococci by a positive litmus milk decolorization reaction (**130**). *Streptococcus milleri* (**131**) is a micro-aerophillic *Streptococcus* associated with abdominal and brain abscesses.

Aerobic Gram-positive Bacilli

The characteristics of Gram-positive bacilli are summarized in **132–134**.

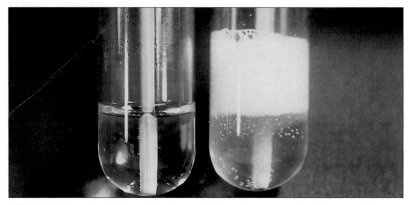

119 Catalase test. Staphylococci (catalase positive) and streptococci (catalase negative) can be distinguished by the catalase test. Catalase-positive organisms break down hydrogen peroxide to oxygen and water. A small inoculum of the bacteria is added to a tube containing 2–3 ml hydrogen peroxide. Active bubbling occurs with catalase-positive organisms. Left, catalase negative; right, catalase positive *(1 min after mixing with H_2O_2).*

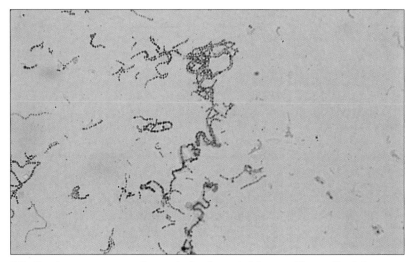

120 *Streptococcus pyogenes*. Gram stain showing typical Gram-positive cocci in chains. Streptococci of different Lancefield groups have a similar Gram appearance. *(Gram stain, ×1000)*

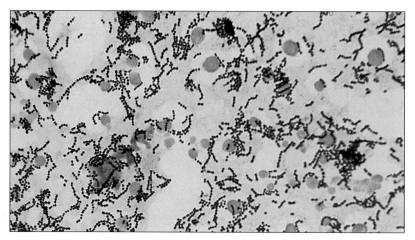

121 *Streptococcus agalactiae* **(Lancefield group B).** Gram stain showing Gram-positive cocci in a blood culture from a neonate. Group B streptococci are an important cause of neonatal sepsis and meningitis. *(Gram stain, ×1000)*

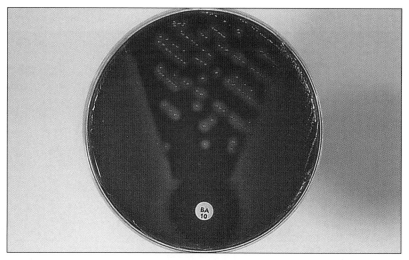

122 *Streptococcus pyogenes* **culture.** Cultured on blood agar, showing beta (clear) zones of hemolysis around the colonies. The plate also contains a bacitracin disk to which *S. pyogenes* (unlike most other beta hemolytic streptococci) is sensitive. *(Blood agar, 18 h at 37ºC)*

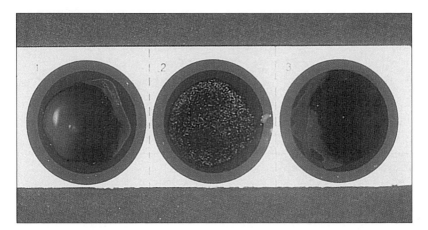

123 Lancefield grouping. Beta hemolytic streptococci are classified into Lancefield groups according to their surface carbohydrate antigens. A slide agglutination test can be used with antisera to the different Lancefield groups. Positive agglutination with the appropriate antisera will determine the group. Positive agglutination in centre circle. *(Agglutination after 2 min at room temperature)*

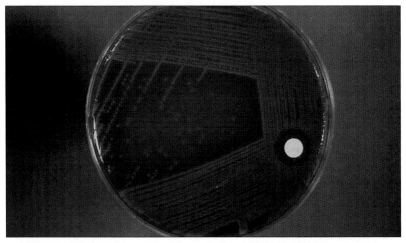

124 *Streptococcus pneumoniae*. Cultured on blood agar. Note the alpha (green) hemolysis and the 'draughtsman' shape of the colonies. The plate contains an optochin disk, to which *S. pneumoniae*, in contrast to other alpha hemolytic streptococci, is sensitive. *(Blood agar, 18 h at 37ºC)*

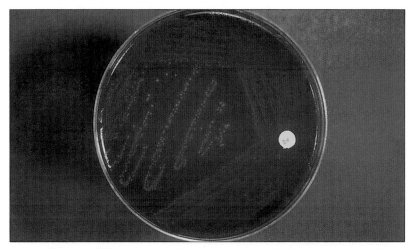

125 *Streptococcus viridans*. Culture on blood agar, showing alpha hemolysis and optochin resistance. Viridans streptococci are normal oral flora but are an important cause of bacterial endocarditis in patients with congenital or acquired abnormalities of the heart valves. *(Blood agar, 18 h at 37°C)*

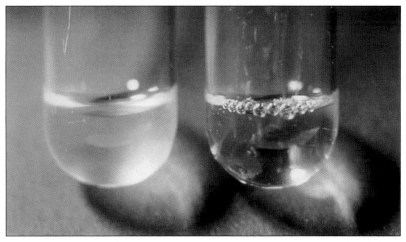

126 Bile solubility test. This is a further test for distinguishing pneumococci from other alpha hemolytic streptococci. A heavy inoculum of the test organism is emulsified in saline and the bile salt sodium deoxycholate added. The bile salt dissolves *S. pneumoniae* and clears the turbidity. Left, *S. viridans*; right, *S. pneumoniae*. *(Solubility demonstrated 3 min after the addition of bile salt)*

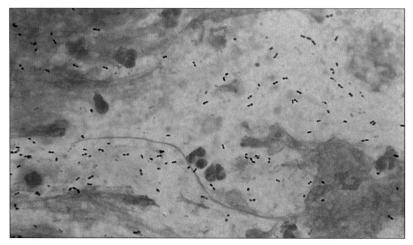

127 *Streptococcus pneumoniae*. Gram stain showing Gram-positive diplococci with a lanceolate shape typical of *S. pneumoniae* (pneumococcus). This is a Gram stain of sputum from a patient with pneumococcal pneumonia. *(Gram stain, ×1000)*

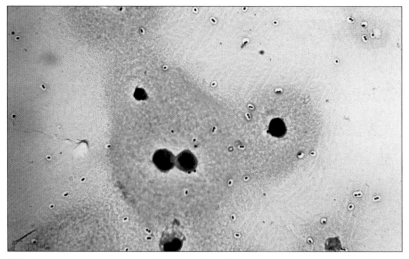

128 *Streptococcus pneumoniae*. Gram stain of the CSF of a patient with pneumococcal meningitis. The clear areas surrounding the diplococci are formed by the capsules. *(Gram, ×1000)*

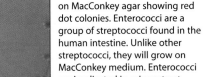

129 *Enterococcus faecalis.* Growth on MacConkey agar showing red dot colonies. Enterococci are a group of streptococci found in the human intestine. Unlike other streptococci, they will grow on MacConkey medium. Enterococci are implicated in urinary tract infections, wound infections and bacterial endocarditis. *(MacConkey agar, 18 h at 37°C)*

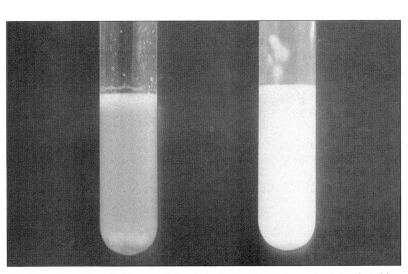

130 *Enterococcus faecalis.* Litmus milk decolorization test. The test organism is incubated for 4 h at 37°C in the litmus milk reagent. Enterococci (right) decolorize the litmus. The negative control is *Streptococcus viridans*. *(4 h at 37°C)*

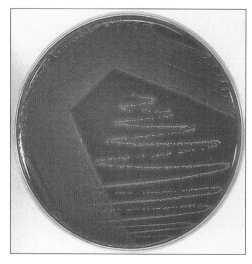

131 *Streptococcus milleri.*
Streptococcus milleri is a commensal in the alimentary tract and is associated with intra-abdominal abscesses. It produces small colonies on blood agar. *(Blood agar, 18 h at 37°C)*

Bacillus spp
Bacillus spp are spore-forming, Gram-positive bacilli. Many are non-pathogenic, but *B. anthracis* is the cause of the disease anthrax. **135** shows anthrax bacilli stained by the McFadyean reaction, and **136** shows *B. anthracis* cultured on blood agar. *Bacillus cereus* is a cause of food poisoning (**137**). It can be cultured on the selective medium mannitol, egg yolk, phenol red, polymyxin agar (**138**).

Listeria spp
Listeria monocytogenes is a cause of infection in neonates and the immunocompromised, and is usually acquired in food. It is a small, Gram-positive bacillus (**139**) and produces pale colonies on blood agar (**140**).

Corynebacteria
Corynebacterium diphtheriae is the cause of diphtheria. Neisser's staining shows the metachromatic volutin granules in diphtheria bacilli (**141**). Gram staining of *Corynebacterium* shows small Gram-positive rods, often arranged as 'Chinese lettering' (**142**). *Corynebacterium diphtheriae* is divided into three biotopes – gravis, intermedius and mitis – all of which produce black colonies on tellurite medium (**143**). There is some variation in the colonial appearance of the different biotopes (**144, 145**). Only toxigenic strains of *C. diphtheriae* cause diphtheria. The Elek test (**146**) is used to demonstrate toxin production.

AEROBIC GRAM-POSITIVE BACILLI INFECTIONS					
Organism	Major infection	Less common infection	Vaccine preventable?	Incubation period	Period of infectivity
(a) Spore forming *Bacillus*					
B. anthracis	Anthrax		(Yes)	2–5 days	–
B. cereus	Food poisoning	Wound infections, endocarditis	No		
(b) Non- spore forming *Listeria*					
L. mono-cytogenes	Neonatal sepsis, meningitis	Septicemia in immuno-compromised	No	3 days – 3 weeks	
Corynebacterium					
C. diphtheriae	Diphtheria	Skin infections	Yes	2–5 days	Up to 4 weeks
C. urealyticum	Cystitis		No		
C. jeikeium	Infection associated with prosthetic devices and intravenous or CSF catheters		No		
Erysipelothrix					
E. rhusiopathiae	Erysipeloid	Bacteremia, endocarditis	No	–	–
Lactobacillus spp	–	Rarely associated with endocarditis, abscesses	No	–	–

132 Aerobic Gram-positive bacilli. Infections.

GRAM-POSITIVE BACILLI
SOURCES AND TRANSMISSION OF BACTERIA

Organism	Man	Animal	Env.	Feco-oral	Droplet	Direct	Nosocomial	Comments
		Reservoir			Transmission			
Bacillus anthracis	–	+	+	–	+	+	–	Category III pathogen
B. cereus	–	–	+	+	–	+	–	
Listeria monocytogenes	+	+	+	+	–	+ (neo-natal)	–	
Corynebacterium diphtheriae	+	–	–	–	+	+	–	Toxin production demonstrated by Elek test
C. urealyticum	+	–	–	–	–	+	–	
C. jeikeium	+	–	–	–	–	+	+	
Erysipelothrix rhusiopathiae	–	+	+		–	+	–	Infections mostly in farm/ veterinary workers
Lactobacillus spp	+	–	–	–	–	+/–	–	

133 Gram-positive bacilli. Sources and transmission of bacteria.

GRAM-POSITIVE BACILLI
IDENTIFYING CHARACTERISTICS

Organism	Gram	Culture	Biochemical and other tests
Bacillus anthracis	Large +ve bacilli	Gray-white on blood agar, non-hemolytic	Red-mauve bacilli on staining with Loeffler's methylene blue, positive gelatin liquefaction
B. cereus	Large +ve bacilli	Beta hemolytic on blood agar	Gray colonies on mannitol, egg yolk, polymyxin agar
Listeria monocytogenes	Small +ve bacilli	Beta hemolytic on blood agar	'Tumbling motility', grows well at 4°C Biochemical differentiation by Hiss' sugars
Corynebacterium diphtheriae	Pleomorphic +ve bacilli Volutin granules demonstrated by Albert's stain	Black colonies on tellurite medium	Glu Mal Suc Starch Urea + + – + –

134 Gram-positive bacilli. Identifying characteristics.

**GRAM-POSITIVE BACILLI
IDENTIFYING CHARACTERISTICS (Cont'd)**

Organism	Gram	Culture	Biochemical and other tests				
			Glu	Mal	Suc	Starch	Urea
C. hofmannii	+ve bacilli	Black colonies on tellurite medium	–	–	–	–	+
C. urealyticum	+ve bacilli	Black colonies on tellurite medium	–	–	–	–	+
C. jeikeium	+ve bacilli	Black colonies on tellurite medium	+	+/–	–	+/–	–
Erysipelothrix rhusiopathiae	Small +ve bacilli	Alpha hemolysis on blood sugar	Non-motile: produces H_2S in triple sugar agar				
Lactobacillus spp	Large +ve bacilli	Variable colony appearance and size	Catalase –ve				

134 Gram-positive bacilli. Identifying characteristics. (*Cont'd*)

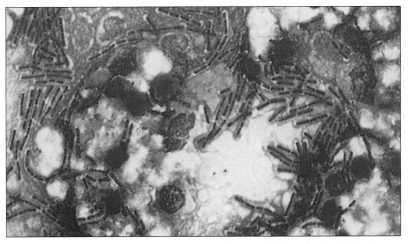

135 *Bacillus anthracis*. Stained with Loeffler's polychrome methylene blue (McFadyean's reaction). The capsule of *B. anthracis* stains red-mauve. (*Polychrome methylene blue, ×1000*)

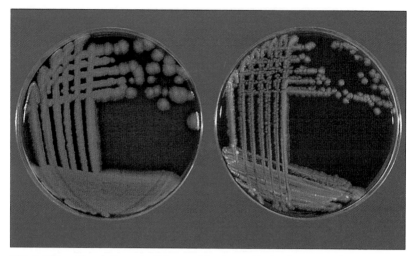

136 Bacillus anthracis/B. cereus. Culture on blood agar, showing large, gray-white colonies with wavy edges. Saprophytic *Bacillus* species are usually hemolytic. Anthrax is highly infectious, and great care must be taken if specimens are processed in the laboratory. *(Blood agar, 18 h at 37°C)*

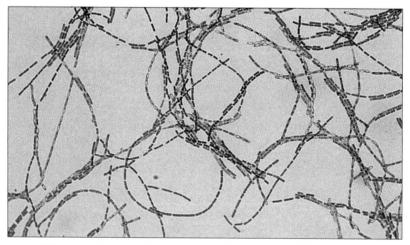

137 Bacillus cereus. Gram stain showing the large, Gram-positive bacilli, often arranged in chains. *Bacillus cereus* is a cause of food poisoning, and a selective medium – mannitol, egg yolk, phenol red, polymyxin agar (MYPA) is used to isolate it from feces or food. *(Gram stain, ×1000)*

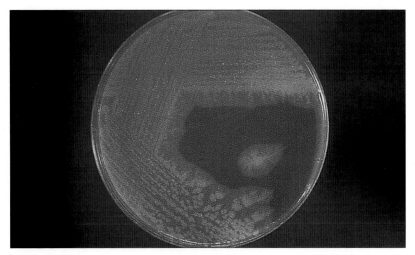

138 *Bacillus cereus*, mannitol, egg yolk, phenol red, polymyxin agar (MYPA). *Bacillus cereus* produces large, gray-white colonies, surrounded by an area of white precipitate. MYPA may be used as a selective medium in the investigation of food poisoning to isolate *B. cereus* from feces or food. *(MYPA, 18 h at 37°C)*

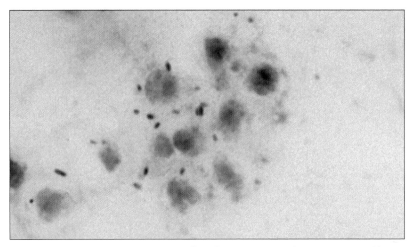

139 *Listeria monocytogenes*. Gram stain of CSF from a neonate with meningitis caused by *L. monocytogenes* showing small, Gram-positive bacilli. *(Gram stain, ×1000)*

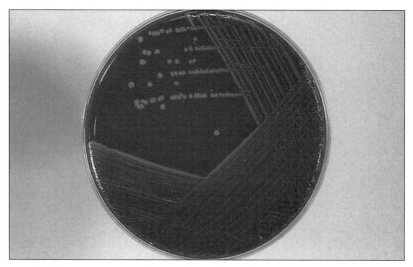

140 *Listeria monocytogenes*. Culture on blood agar, showing small, pale colonies with a zone of beta hemolysis. *Listeria monocytogenes* can grow at 4°C. *(Blood agar, 18 h at 37°C)*

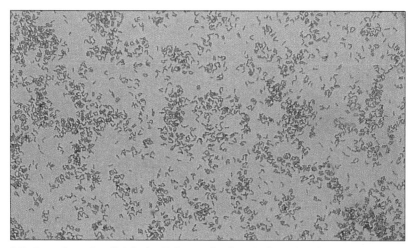

141 *Corynebacterium diphtheriae*, Neisser stain. The stain shows the volutin granules within the bacilli, which are characteristic of *C. diphtheriae*. *(Neisser stain, ×1000)*

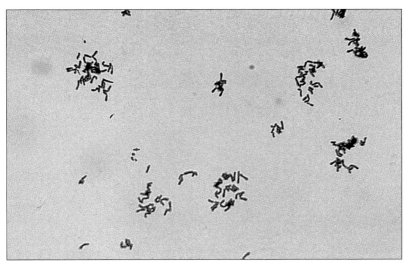

142 Gram stain of diphtheroids. The term 'diphtheroids' includes various *Corynebacterium* species that are skin commensals. The Gram stain shows a typical 'Chinese lettering' arrangement of the bacilli. *(Gram stain, ×1000)*

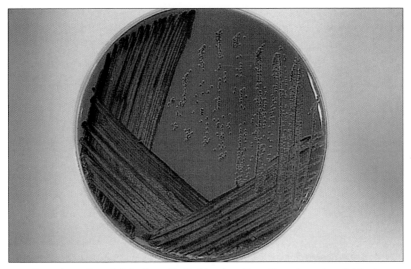

143 *Corynebacterium diphtheriae*, tellurite blood medium. *Corynebacterium diphtheriae* reduces tellurite and produces gray-black colonies. Commensal diphtheroids are gray. *(Tellurite blood agar, 48 h at 37ºC)*

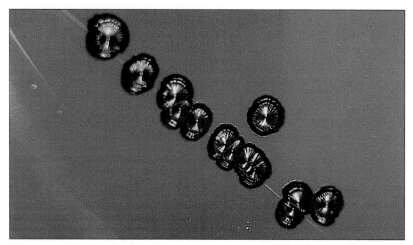

144 *Corynebacterium diphtheriae*, **gravis type.** Close-up of colonies showing striated margins (daisy head appearance). *(Tellurite blood agar, 48 h at 37ºC)*

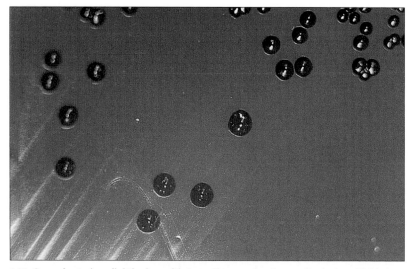

145 *Corynebacterium diphtheriae*, **mitis type.** Close-up showing small colonies with black centres. *(Tellurite blood agar, 48 h at 37ºC)*

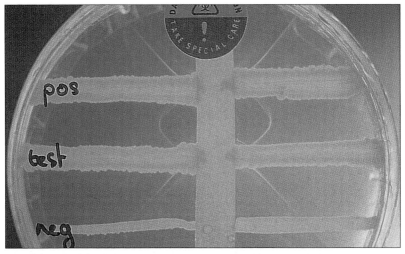

146 Elek plate to demonstrate the toxigenicity of *Corynebacterium diphtheriae*. The filter paper strip contains diphtheria antitoxin; it is placed in the Petri dish and the medium is poured on. The test strain and toxigenic and non-toxigenic strains are inoculated at right angles to the strip. A toxigenic strain produces a V-shaped line of precipitation between the toxin and anti-toxin. *(Elek's medium, 48 h at 37°C)*

Several corynebacteria are non-pathogenic (**147**), and these can be differentiated from C. *diphtheriae* by biochemical tests, using Hiss's serum sugars (**148–150**). Some 'diphtheroids', now designated C. *jeikeium*, are a cause of bacteremia associated with intravenous catheters.

Lactobacilli
Lactobacilli (**151, 152**) are part of the normal flora of the alimentary tract and vagina, and are rarely associated with disease. They are increasingly used in probiotic supplements.

■ AEROBIC GRAM-NEGATIVE BACTERIA
Aerobic Gram-negative Bacilli
Enterobacteriaceae
The characteristics of this family are summarized in **153–157**.

The Enterobacteriaceae comprise a wide range of species, including intestinal commensal bacteria and important pathogens such as *Shigella* and *Salmonella*. Gram staining cannot differentiate between the different *Enterobacteriaceae*. **158** shows the typical appearance; in this case, it is *Escherichia coli*. Enterobacteria (coliforms) will all grow on MacConkey medium, which can distinguish lactose-fermenting (pink) from non-lactose-fermenting (pale) species.

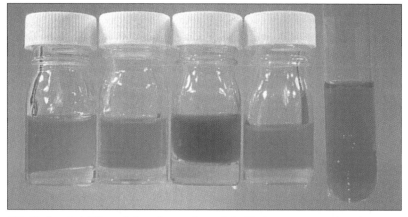

147 *Corynebacterium hofmannii.* Close-up of colonies showing the raised, cone-shaped appearance. *(Tellurite blood agar, 24 h at 37ºC)*

148 Biochemical differentiation of corynebacteria by Hiss' serum sugars. The tubes contain from left to right glucose, maltose, sucrose, starch and urea. *Corynebacterium diphtheriae gravis* produces acid from glucose, maltose and starch. *(Hiss' serum water sugars with phenol red indicator, 24 h at 37ºC)*

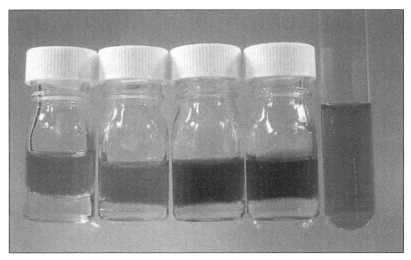

149 Biochemical differentiation of corynebacteria by Hiss' serum sugars. *Corynebacterium diphtheriae mitis* is positive for glucose and maltose.

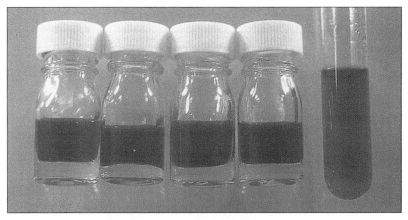

150 Biochemical differentiation of corynebacteria by Hiss' serum sugars. *Corynebacterium hofmannii*, a throat commensal, does not ferment the sugars, but is urease positive.

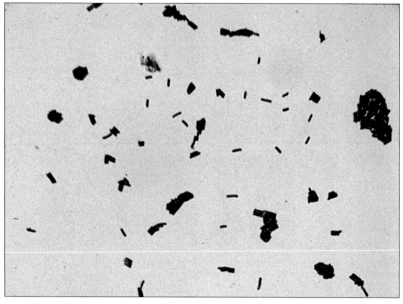

151 Gram stain of lactobacilli. Lactobacilli are large, Gram-positive rods that occur singly and in chains. They are part of the normal vaginal flora. *(Gram stain, ×1000)*

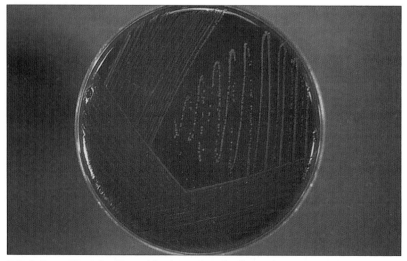

152 Culture of *Lactobacillus* on blood agar. Lactobacilli grow best in a 5% carbon dioxide atmosphere, producing small, pale colonies. *(Blood agar, 18 h at 37°C)*

ENTEROBACTERIACEAE INFECTIONS

Organism	Major infection	Less common infection	Vaccine preventables	Incubation period	Period of infectivity
Escherichia					
E. coli	Urinary tract, wound infection, septicemia, neonatal meningitis	Gastroenteritis by some serotypes	–	–	–
Klebsiella					
K. oxytoca	Urinary tract	Septicemia	–	–	–
K. pneumoniae	Urinary tract, chest infections	Septicemia			
K. granulomatis	Genital lesions (Donovanosis)				
Enterobacter					
E. cloacae	Wound, urinary tract	Septicemia	–	–	–
E. aerogenes			–	–	–
Shigella					
S. dysenteriae	Bacillary dysentery	–	–	3–4 days	
S. flexneri	Bacillary dysentery	–	–	3–4 days	1–4 weeks
S. boydii	Bacillary dysentery	–	–	3–4 days	
S. sonnei	Bacillary dysentery	–	–	3–4 days	
Salmonella					
S. typhi	Typhoid fever	Osteomyelitis	+	7–21 days	Variable, 5–21 days
S. paratyphi A	Paratyphoid fever		+/–	7–21 days	Some long-term excreters
S. paratyphi B	Paratyphoid fever	Septicemia	+/–	7–21 days	
S. typhimurium[a]	Gastroenteritis	Osteomyelitis	–	1–3 days	

[a]*S. typhimurium* is given as the example of a large number of non-typhi salmonella serotypes.

153 Enterobacteriaceae. Infections.

ENTEROBACTERIACEAE INFECTIONS					
Organism	Major infection	Less common infection	Vaccine preventable?	Incubation period	Period of infectivity
Citrobacter C. freundii	Urinary tract, wound infections	Septicemia	–	–	–
Edwardsiella E. tarda	Wound infection		–	–	–
Serratia S. marcescens	Wound infection	Septicemia	–	–	–
Hafnia H. alvei	–	Rarely urinary tract infection, septicemia	–	–	–
Proteus P. mirabilis	Urinary tract, wound infection	Septicemia	–	–	–
P. vulgaris	Urinary tract, wound infection		–	–	–
Morganella M. morganii	Urinary tract, burns infections		–	–	–
Yersinia Y. enterocolitica	Gastroenteritis		–	–	–
Y. pseudo-tuberculosis	Mesenteric adenitis	Septicemia, pneumonia	–	–	–
Y. pestis	Bubonic plague (rat plague)		Killed vaccine available	1–6 days	see **156**

154 Enterobacteriaceae. Infections.

ENTEROBACTERIACEAE
SOURCES AND TRANSMISSION OF BACTERIA

Organism	Reservoir			Transmission				Comments
	Man	Animal	Env.	Feco-oral	Droplet	Direct	Nosocomial	
Escherichia coli	+	+	+	+	−	+	+	
Klebsiella oxytoca	+	−	+	−	−	+	+	
K. pneumoniae	+	−	+	−	+	+	+	
Enterobacter cloacae	+	−	+	−	−	+	+	
E. aerogenes	+	−	+	−	−	+	+	Large epidemics of multiply antimicrobial-resistant strains may occur
Shigella dysenteriae	+	−	−	+	−	−	−	
S. flexneri	+	−	−	+	−	−	−	
S. boydii	+	−	−	+	−	−	−	
S. sonnei	+	−	−	+	−	−	−	
Salmonella typhi	+	−	−	+	−	−	−	
S. paratyphi A	+	−	−	+	−	−	−	
S. paratyphi B	+	+	−	+	−	−	−	
S. typhimurium	+	+	−	+	−	−	−	

155 Enterobacteriaceae. Sources and transmission of bacteria.

ENTEROBACTERIACEAE
SOURCES AND TRANSMISSION OF BACTERIA

Organism	Reservoir			Transmission					Comments
	Man	Animal	Env.	Insect	Feco-oral	Droplet	Direct	Nosocomial	
Citrobacter freundii	+	−	+	−	−	−	+	+	
Edwardsiella tarda	+	−	+	−	−	−	+	+	
Serratia marcescens	+	−	+	−	−	−	+	+	
Hania alvei	+	−	+	−	−	−	+	+	
Proteus mirabilis	+	−	+	−	−	−	+	+	
P. vulgaris	+	−	+	−	−	−	+	+	
Providencia stuartii	+	−	+	−	−	−	+	+	
Morganella morganii	+	−	+	−	−	−	+	+	
Yersinia enterocolitica	+	+	−	−	+	−	−	−	
Y. pseudotuberculosis	+	+	−	−	+	−	−	−	
Y. pestis	+	+	−	+	−	+	−	−	Pneumonic form directly transmissible

156 Enterobacteriaceae. Sources and transmission of bacteria.

ENTEROBACTERIACEAE
BIOCHEMICAL CHARACTERIZATION

	Lac	Gluc	Man	Suc	Cit	Dulc	Ind	Urea	Motile	H₂S	MR[b]	VP[c]	PD[d]	NO₃
Escherichia coli	+	+g[a]	+	+/-	-	+/-	+	-	+	-	+	-	-	+
Klebsiella oxytoca	+	+g	+	+	+	+/-	+	+	-	-	-	+	-	+
K. pneumoniae	+	+g	+	+	+	+/-	-	+	-	-	-	+	-	+
Enterobacter cloacae	+	+g	+	+	+	-	-	+/-	+	-	-	+	-	+
E. aerogenes	+	+g	+	+	+	-	-	-	+	-	-	+	-	+
Shigella dysenteriae	-	+	+	-	-	-	+/-	-	-	-	+	-	-	+
S. sonnei	+/-	+	+	-	-	-	-	-	-	-	+	-	-	+
Salmonella typhi	-	+	+	-	-	-	-	-	+	+	+	-	-	+
S. paratyphi A	-	+g	+	-	-	-	-	-	+	-	+	-	-	+
S. paratyphi B	-	?	+	-	-	+	-	-	+	+	+	-	-	+
S. typhimurium	-	+g	+	-	+	+/-	-	-	+	+	+	-	-	+
Citrobacter freundii	-	+g	+	+/-	+	+/-	-	+/-	+	+	+	-	-	+
Edwardsiella tarda	-	+g	-	-	-	-	+	-	+	+	+	-	-	+
Serratia marcescens	-	+/-/g	+	+	+	-	-	-	+	-	-	+	-	+
Hafnia alvei	-	+g	+	-	+	-	-	-	+	-	+/-	+/-	-	+
Proteus mirabilis	-	+g	-	+/-	+/-	-	-	+	+	+	+	-	+	+
P. vulgaris	-	+g	-	+	+/-	-	+	+	+	+	+	-	+	+
Providencia stuartii	-	+g	-	+/-	+	-	+	+/-	+	-	+	-	+	+
Morganella morganii	-	+g	-	-	-	-	+/-	+	+	-	+	-	+	+
Yersinia enterocolitica	-	+	+	+	-	-	-	+/-	-	-	+	-	-	+
Y. pseudotuberculosis	-	+	+	-	-	-	-	+	-	-	+	-	-	+
Y. pestis	-	+	+	-	-	-	-	-	-	-	+	-	-	+

ᵃGas production. ᵇMethyl red. ᶜVoges–Proskauer. ᵈPhenylalanine deaminase.

157 Enterobacteriaceae. Biochemical characterization.

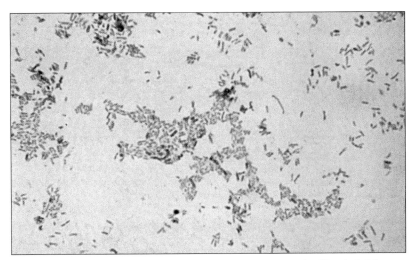

158 *Escherichia coli,* **Gram stain.** The stain shows the Gram-negative bacilli typical of the Enterobacteriaceae. Most have a similar morphology and cannot be distinguished by Gram staining. *(Gram stain, ×1000)*

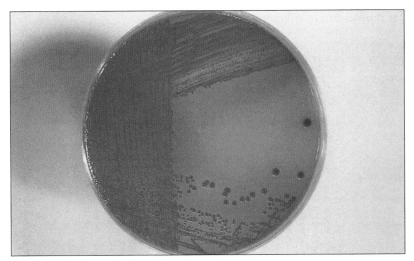

159 *Escherichia coli,* **MacConkey medium.** *Escherichia coli* produces pink, lactose-fermenting colonies. MacConkey medium is a selective medium for enteric bacteria, containing bile salts, lactose and the pH indicator neutral red. Lactose-fermenting colonies produce acid and turn the indicator red. *(MacConkey agar, 18 h at 37ºC)*

159 shows the lactose-fermenting *E. coli* cultured on MacConkey medium, and **160** the pale, non-lactose-fermenting colonies of *Proteus mirabilis*. **161** shows the mucoid lactose-fermenting colonies of *Klebsiella pneumoniae*. **162** shows the differentiation between coliform bacteria (larger green-blue colonies) and staphylococci (smaller, white colonies) from a urine sample grown on cystine, lactose, electrolyte-deficient (CLED) medium. MacConkey medium containing sorbitol in place of lactose can be used to distinguish the *E. coli* serotype O157 that causes hemorrhagic colitis from other *E. coli*. *Escherichia coli* O157 does not ferment sorbitol and forms pale colonies on sorbitol MacConkey (**163, 164**). *Proteus* spp have the characteristic of 'swarming' when cultured on blood agar (**165**) but this is inhibited by bile (**160**).

166 shows lactose-fermenting *E. coli* and non-lactose-fermenting *Shigella sonnei* cultured on MacConkey medium. More selective media such as xylose lysine desoxycholate (XLD) may be used to isolate *Shigella* or *Salmonella* from fecal specimens (**167, 168**). Other selective media for these species include *Salmonella–Shigella* (SS) agar and deoxycholate citrate agar (DCA) (**169, 170**).

A wide range of sugar fermentation and other biochemical tests may be used to differentiate between the different Enterobacteriaceae. **171–175** show examples of sugar fermentation reactions using peptone-water sugars. **176** shows the tube indole test that can distinguish between *E. coli* and *K. pneumoniae*. **177–181** show other biochemical tests commonly used in the differentiation of Enterobacteriaceae.

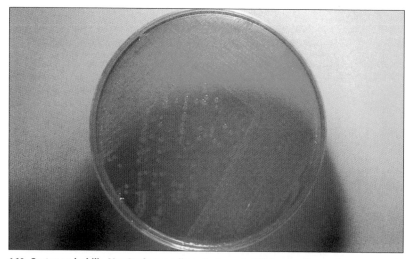

160 *Proteus mirabilis*, MacConkey medium. *Proteus mirabilis* is a non-lactose fermenter and produces pale colonies on MacConkey medium. *(MacConkey agar, 18 h at 37ºC)*

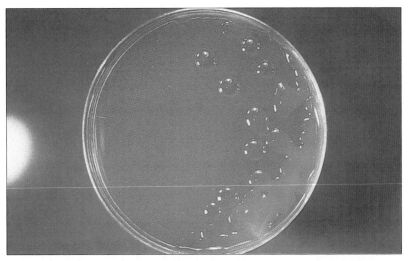

161 *Klebsiella pneumoniae*, **MacConkey medium.** *Klebsiella pneumoniae* is a lactose fermenter and produces pink, mucoid colonies. *(MacConkey agar, 18 h at 37ºC)*

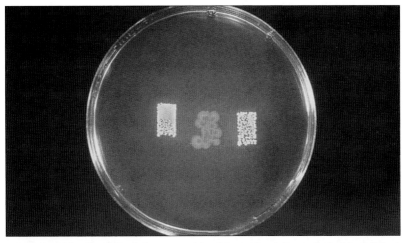

162 *Escherichia coli* and *Staphylococcus epidermidis*, **cystine, lactose, electrolyte-deficient (CLED) medium.** CLED agar is used as a selective medium for urine samples. *Escherichia coli* produces large colonies with a bluish color; *S. epidermidis* produces small, white colonies. *(CLED agar, 18 h at 37ºC)*

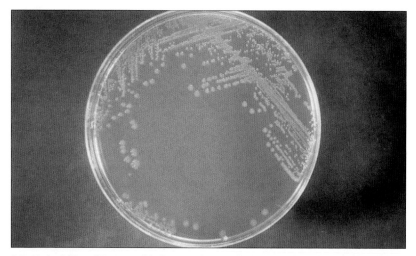

163 *Escherichia coli* O157, sorbitol MacConkey medium. *Escherichia coli* serogroup O157 is an important pathogen causing hemorrhagic colitis and hemolytic uremic syndrome. It does not ferment sorbitol and produces pale colonies on MacConkey medium in which lactose is replaced by sorbitol. *(Sorbitol MacConkey agar, 18 h at 37ºC)*

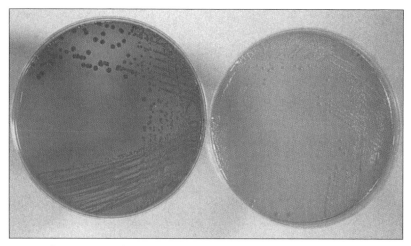

164 *E. coli* O157, MacConkey and sorbitol MacConkey. *Escherichia coli* O157 is a lactose fermenter and produces pink colonies on standard MacConkey agar (left), compared with the non-sorbitol fermenters on the selective medium (right). *(MacConkey and sorbitol MacConkey agar, 18 h at 37ºC)*

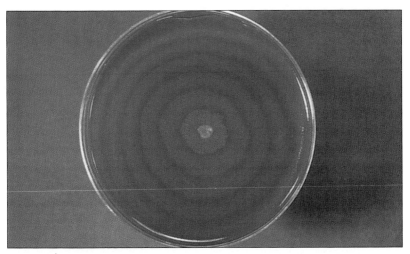

165 *Proteus mirabilis*, **blood agar.** *Proteus mirabilis* produces swarming growth on blood agar that may often conceal other bacteria in a mixed growth. *(Blood agar, 18 h at 37°C)*

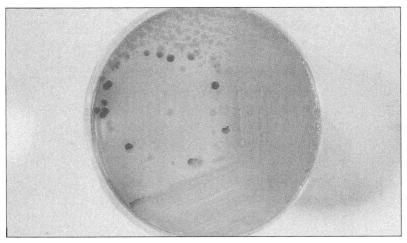

166 *Escherichia coli* and *Shigella sonnei*, **MacConkey medium.** *Shigella* colonies are pale, are non-lactose fermenting and often have a characteristic wavy edge. *Escherichia coli* shows the typical pink, lactose-fermenting colonies. *(MacConkey agar, 18 h at 37°C)*

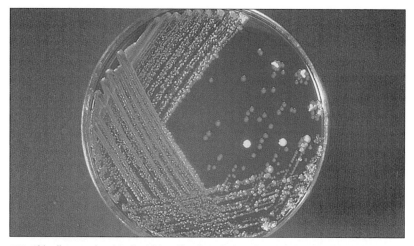

167 *Shigella sonnei* and *Escherichia coli*, xylose, lysine, deoxycholate (XLD) medium. XLD is a selective medium for the isolation of *Shigella* and *Salmonella* from fecal specimens. XLD contains the indicator phenol red, which is red at alkaline pH and yellow at acid pH. *Shigella* forms red colonies as it does not ferment xylose; *E. coli* produces pale yellow colonies. *(XLD medium, 18 h at 37ºC)*

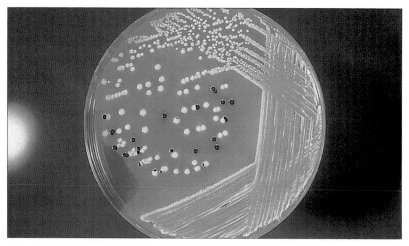

168 *Salmonella enteritidis* and *Escherichia coli*, xylose, lysine, deoxycholate (XLD) medium. *Salmonella* produces red colonies with black centers from hydrogen sulfide production. *Escherichia coli* forms yellow colonies. *(XLD medium, 18 h at 37ºC)*

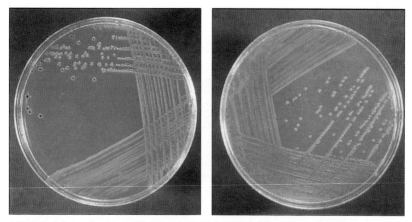

169, 170 *Salmonella enteritidis, Salmonella/Shigella* **(SS) agar (169) and deoxycholate, citrate agar (DCA, 170).** SS agar and DCA are also selective media for isolating these pathogens from fecal specimens. On both, *Salmonella* produce pale, non-lactose-fermenting colonies. *(SS agar and DCA, 18 h at 37ºC)*

REACTIONS IN PEPTONE-WATER SUGARS						
Code:	**Glucose – green**	**Mannite – purple**	**Lactose – red**	**Sucrose – blue**	**Dulcite – pink**	**Urea – black**
Escherichia coli	A G	A G	A G	– –	– –	–
Shigella sonnei	A –	A –	– –	– –	– –	–
Salmonella typhimurium	A G	A G	– –	– –	A G	–
Proteus mirabilis	A G	– –	– –	– –	– –	+
A = acid production (pink). G = gas production (bubbles in tube).						

171 Reactions in peptone-water sugars.

172–175 Peptone-water sugar reactions of Enterobacteriaceae. A series of peptone-water sugars – glucose, mannite, lactose, sucrose, dulcite and urea – can be used for the biochemical differentiation of the Enterobacteriaceae. Acid production changes the indicator to red, gas production being shown by bubbles in the inverted tube. *(Peptone-water sugars, Andrade's indicator, 24 h at 37°C)*

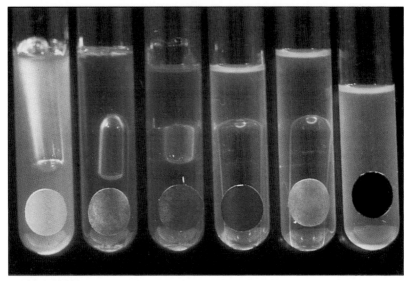

172 *Escherichia coli.*

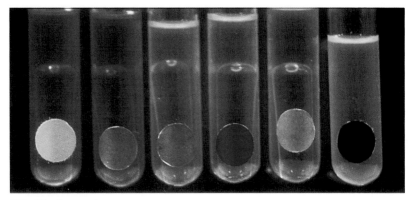

173 *Shigella sonnei.*

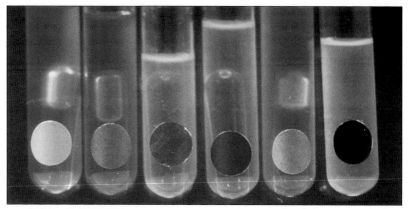

174 *Salmonella typhimurium.*

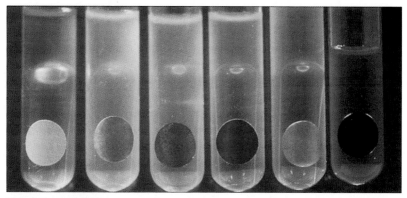

175 *Proteus mirabilis.*

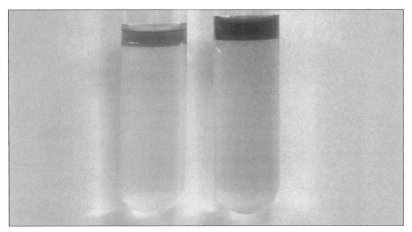

176 Tube indole test. Indole-positive bacteria break down the amino acid tryptophan to indole, which reacts with Kovac's reagent to produce a red color. *Escherichia coli*, indole positive (right); *Klebsiella pneumoniae*, indole negative (left). *(Peptone-water, 24 h at 37°C)*

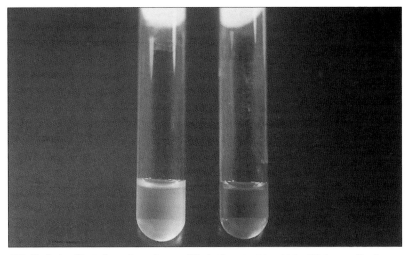

177 Methyl red test. Enterobacteriaceae differ in the extent to which pH is lowered in glucose fermentation. With methyl red indicator, only those which reduce the pH to approximately 5 will change the indicator to a red color. *Escherichia coli*, methyl red positive (right); *Enterobacter aerogenes*, methyl red negative (left). *(Glucose phosphate/peptone-water, 24 h at 37°C)*

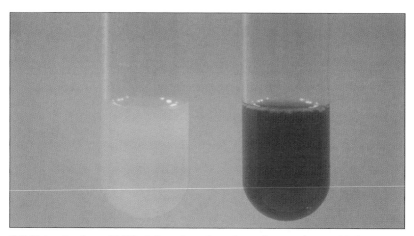

178 Voges-Proskauer (V-P) test. Some Enterobacteriaceae ferment glucose with the production of acetyl methylcarbinol, which is oxidized and reacts with alpha-naphthol to produce a red color. *Enterobacter aerogenes,* V-P positive (right); *Escherichia coli,* V-P negative (left). *(Glucose phosphate/peptone-water, 48 h at 37ºC, alpha-naphthol and KOH added and viewed after 5 min)*

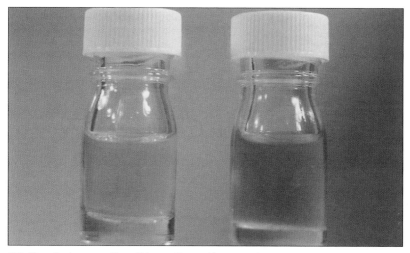

179 Koser's citrate medium. This test distinguishes Enterobacteriaceae that can utilize citrate as the sole source of carbon. The indicator bromothymol blue turns from green to blue as a result of the alkaline reaction. *Citrobacter freundii,* positive (right); *Escherichia coli,* negative (left). *(Koser's citrate medium, 18 h at 37ºC)*

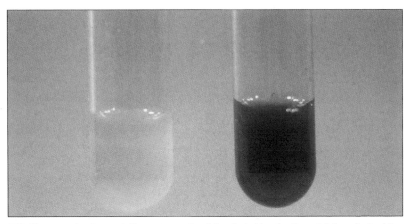

180 Nitrate reduction test. The test organism is incubated in a broth containing nitrate. After 4 h, the broth is tested for the reduction of nitrate to nitrite, which reacts to form a red color with sulfanilic acid and alpha-naphthylamine. *Escherichia coli*, positive nitrate reduction (right); *Ps. aeruginosa*, negative nitrate reduction (left). *(Nitrate broth, 4 h at 37°C)*

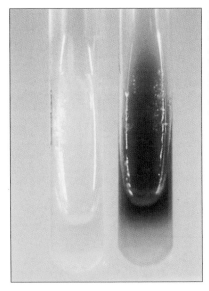

181 Phenylalanine deaminase test. Certain Enterobacteriaceae (*Proteus*, *Providencia*) break down phenylalanine to produce phenylpyruvic acid, which gives a green-brown color with ferric chloride. *Proteus mirabilis*, phenylalanine positive (right); *Escherichia coli*, phenylalanine negative (left). *(Phenylalanine agar, 18 h at 37°C; then four drops 10% w/v ferric chloride added and observe after 5 min)*

Combinations of these tests are now available in a variety of commercial systems, examples being shown in **182** and **183**. These systems have now been automated so they can be read and interpreted using computerized databases (**184**).

Where resources are limited, particularly in developing countries, biochemical differentiation can be achieved by using inexpensive composite media. **185–187** show Kligler iron agar composite medium, and **188–190** motility-indole-urea medium, used to distinguish the pathogens *Shigella* and *Salmonella* from other enterobacteria. *Salmonella* spp include the causes of typhoid and paratyphoid fevers, as well as a large number of serotypes responsible for less severe gastrointestinal disease. The serotypes are distinguished by their O (somatic) and H (flagella) antigens (the Kauffman–White typing scheme). **191** shows a slide agglutination test to determine the *Salmonella* O serotypes, using specific O antisera.

Typhoid and paratyphoid fevers may also be diagnosed by identifying specific O and H antibodies in the patient's serum using the Widal test (**192, 193**). Dilutions of the serum are incubated with standard H and O suspensions of *S. typhi* or *S. paratyphi* and the highest titres (reciprocal dilutions) read for H flocculation and O agglutination determined. The Enterobacteriaceae also contain the species *Yersinia*, which includes the cause of plague, *Y. pestis* (**194**), and *Y. enterocolitica*, causing mesenteric adenitis and enterocolitis (**195**).

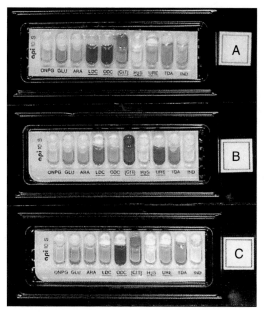

182 API-10S kit for Enterobacteriaceae. These kits use dried reagents in cupules to which a suspension of the test organisms is added. The strips are incubated overnight and the reactions determined. This allows the rapid processing of a large number of isolates. Tests in strips from left to right are: ONPG, GLU, ARA, LDC, ODC, CIT, H_2S, UREA, TDA, INDOLE, NO_2. **A** *Escherichia coli*. **B** *Klebsiella pneumoniae*. **C** *Shigella sonnei*. (API-10S kits, 18 h at 37ºC)

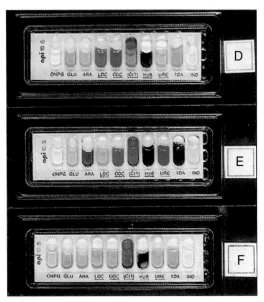

183 API-10S diagnostic strips (cont.). D *Salmonella typhimurium.* **E** *Proteus mirabilis.* **F** *Citrobacter freundi.* (API-10S kits, 18 h at 37°C)

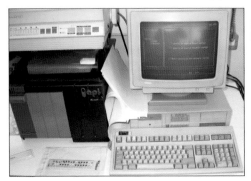

184 Automated reader of biochemical bacterial identification strips.

REACTIONS IN KLIGLER IRON AGAR

	Base (glucose fermentation) if yellow	Slope (lactose fermentation) if yellow	Gas production	H₂S production
Before culture	Pink	Pink	–	–
Escherichia coli	Yellow	Yellow	+	–
Shigella sonnei	Yellow	Pink	–	–
Salmonella enteritidis	Yellow-black	Pink-black	+/–	+
Proteus mirabilis	Yellow-black	Pink-black	+	+

185 Reactions in Kligler iron agar.

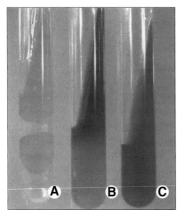

186 Enterobacteriaceae reactions in Kligler iron agar (KIA). KIA is a composite medium containing glucose, lactose, phenol red and ferric citrate. A yellow base indicates glucose fermentation, whereas a yellow base and a slope indicate both glucose and lactose fermentation. Bubbles in the medium show gas production from glucose. Blackening of the medium indicates hydrogen sulfide production. **A** *Escherichia coli*. **B** *Shigella sonnei*. **C** Uninoculated. *(KIA, 18 h at 37ºC)*

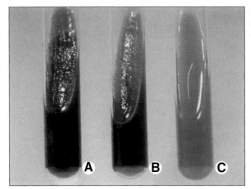

187 Kligler iron agar. A *Salmonella enteritidis*. **B** *Proteus mirabilis*. **C** Uninoculated. *(KIA, 18 h at 37ºC)*

REACTIONS IN MOTILITY-INDOLE-UREA MEDIUM			
	Motility	**Indole**	**Urea**
Escherichia coli	+	+	–
Shigella sonnei	–	–/+	–
Salmonella enteritidis	+	–	–
Proteus mirabilis	+	–	+

188 Reactions in motility-indole-urea medium.

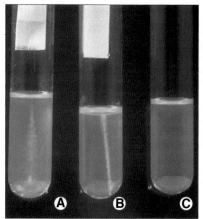

189 Enterobacteriaceae reactions in motility-indole-urea (MIU) medium. MIU is a composite medium containing tryptone, phenol red, urea and a paper strip moistened in Kovac's reagent. It is inoculated by a straight wire through the center of the medium. Non-motile organisms (e.g. *Shigella*) grow only in the line of the inoculum, but motile organisms (most Salmonellae) grow throughout the medium, which becomes turbid. Urease-positive organisms (e.g. *Proteus* spp) turn the medium red. Indole-positive organisms (e.g. *Escherichia coli*) turn the Kovac's strip red. **A** *E. coli*. **B** *Sh. sonnei*. **C** Uninoculated. *(MIU agar, 18 h at 37ºC)*

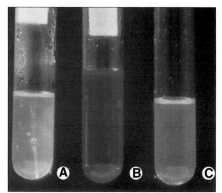

190 Enterobacteriaceae reactions in motility-indole-urea (MIU). **A** *Salmonella enteritidis*. **B** *Proteus mirabilis*. **C** Uninoculated. *(MIU agar, 18 h at 37ºC)*

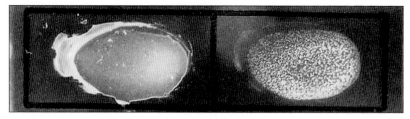

191 *Salmonella* identification by O serotyping. A presumptive *Salmonella* isolate (from culture and biochemical testing) is tested for its O and H antigen type. For O agglutination, an emulsion of the isolate is prepared in saline on a slide and a drop of specific O antiserum added. After 30 seconds, the mixture is observed for visible clumping. *(Agglutination after 30 seconds)*

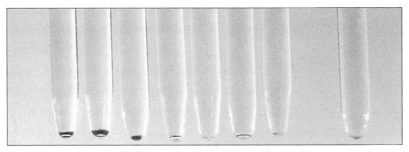

192 Widal test for serological diagnosis of typhoid fever. The Widal test measures the patient's antibodies against *Salmonella typhi* O and H antigen preparations. Serial dilutions of the patient's serum are added to the antigens in tubes, the highest dilution giving granular agglutination with the O antigen and floccular agglutination with the H antigen being reported. Dilutions 1:20–1:1280 and a negative control. O titre 1:80. *(Incubated for 2 h at 37ºC)*

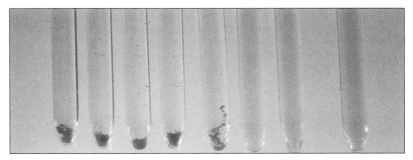

193 Widal test, H agglutination. H titre 1:320. *(Incubated for 3 h at 37ºC)*

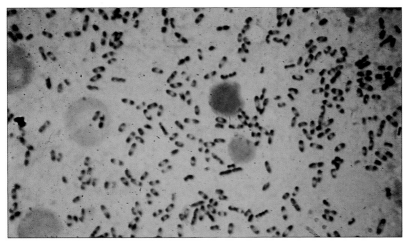

194 *Yersinia pestis* (the plague bacillus), Wayson's stain. Wayson's staining shows coccobacilli with bipolar staining. *(Wayson's stain, ×1000)*

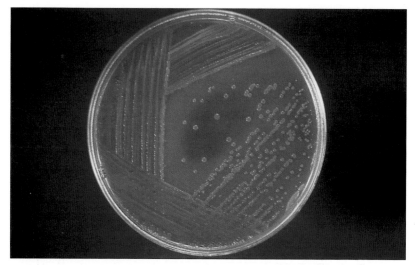

195 *Yersinia enterocolitica*, **cefsoludin, irgasan, novobiocin (CIN) medium.** CIN medium is a selective medium for isolating *Y. enterocolitica* from feces. After 48 h incubation, *Y. enterocolitica* appears as pink colonies with a red center. *(CIN agar, 48 h at 37°C)*

Gram-negative Cocci and Cocco-bacilli

These are summarized in **196–204**.

Neisseria spp

Neisseria spp include the two important pathogens – *N. meningitidis* and *N. gonorrhoeae* – as well as commensal organisms such as *N. lactamica*. **205** is a Gram stain of the CSF fluid from a patient with meningococcal meningitis, showing the paired Gram-negative cocci of *N. meningitidis*. **206** shows colonies of *N. meningitidis* cultured on heated blood ('chocolate') agar. The Gram stain and culture of *N. gonorrhoeae* are shown in **207** and **208**. Selective enriched media, such as modified New York City (MNYC) medium incubated in 5% carbon dioxide in air are necessary to isolate *N. gonorrhoeae* from clinical specimens. *Neisseria* spp are oxidase positive (**209**) and can be distinguished from each other by carbohydrate utilization tests (**210–212**). *Moraxella catarrhalis* (formerly *N. catarrhalis*) is a cause of respiratory infections (**213**). *Moraxella lacunata* (**214**) is a cause of conjunctivitis.

Bordetella spp

Bordetella pertussis, the cause of whooping cough, occurs as Gram-negative cocco-bacilli (**215**).

GRAM-NEGATIVE COCCI AND COCCO-BACILLI INFECTIONS

Organism	Major infection	Less common infection	Vaccine preventable?	Incubation period	Period of infectivity
Neisseria					
N. meningitidis (13 serogroups)	Meningitis, septicemia	Arthritis	Yes (serogroups A/C)	2–10 days	24 h after rifampicin prophylaxis
N. gonorrhoeae	Gonorrhea, pelvic inflammatory disease	Arthritis, conjunctivitis	No	2–7 days	Months if untreated
Moraxella					
M. catarrhalis	Pneumonia	Conjunctivitis, otitis media	No	–	–
M. lacunata	Conjunctivitis	–	No	–	–
Francisella					
F. tularensis	Tularemia	–	Yes	2–10 days	Not directly transmitted

196 Gram-negative cocci and cocco-bacilli. Infections.

GRAM-NEGATIVE COCCI AND COCCO-BACILLI SOURCES AND TRANSMISSION OF BACTERIA

Organism	Reservoir			Transmission					Comments
	Man	Animal	Env.	Insect	Feco-oral	Droplet	Direct	Nosocomial	
Neisseria meningitidis	+	–	–	–	–	+	–	–	Epidemics of serogroup A occur in Africa
N. gonnorrhoeae	+	–	–	–	–	–	+	–	Penicillin-resistant strains increasing
Moraxella catarrhalis	+	–	–	–	–	+	–	–	
M. lacunata	+	–	–	–	–	–	+	–	
Francisella tularensis	–	+	+	+	+	+	+	–	Category III pathogen

197 Gram-negative cocci and cocco-bacilli. Sources and transmission of bacteria.

GRAM-NEGATIVE COCCI AND COCCO-BACILLI IDENTIFYING CHARACTERISTICS

Organism	Gram stain	Culture on blood agar	Oxidase	Biochemical tests
Neisseria meningitidis	–ve diplococci	Gray colonies	+	Ferment glucose and maltose
N. gonorrhoeae	–ve diplococci	No growth	+	Ferment maltose
Moraxella catarrhalis	–ve diplococci	White colonies	+	DNAase +ve
M. lacunata	–ve cocco-bacilli	Poor growth: culture on Dorset egg medium	+	Do not ferment glucose
Francisella tularensis	–ve cocco-bacillus	No growth	–	Identification by agglutination

198 Gram-negative cocci and cocco-bacilli. Identifying characteristics.

GRAM-NEGATIVE COCCO-BACILLI INFECTIONS

Organism	Major infection	Less common infection	Vaccine preventable	Incubation period	Period of infectivity
Acinetobacter					
A. calcaoaceticus	Wound infections, bacteremia	Pneumonia	No	–	–
Bordetella					
B. pertussis	Pertussis (whooping cough)	–	Yes	7–21 days	21 days
B. parapertussis	Parapertussis		No	–	–
Haemophilus					
H. influenzae (type b)	Meningitis, epiglottis, pneumonia, otitis media	Arthritis, osteomyelitis	Yes	2–4 days	In acute stage
H. influenzae (non-capsulated)	Bronchitis, otitis media		No	–	–
H. parainfluenzae	Acute respiratory infections		No	–	–
H. aegyptius	Conjunctivitis, Brazilian hemorrhagic fever		No	–	–
H. ducreyi	Chancroid (venereal infection)		No	3–14 days	1–3 weeks

199 Gram-negative cocco-bacilli. Infections.

GRAM-NEGATIVE COCCO-BACILLI
SOURCES AND TRANSMISSION OF BACTERIA

Organism	Reservoir			Transmission				Comments
	Man	Animal	Env.	Feco-oral	Droplet	Direct	Nosocomial	
Acinetobacter calcaoaceticus	+	–	+	–	+	+	+	
Bordetella pertussis	+	–	–	–	+	–	–	
B. parapertussis	+	–	–	–	+	–	–	
Haemophilus influenzae b	+	–	–	–	+	–	–	
H. influenzae	+	–	–	–	+	–	–	
H. parainfluenzae	+	–	–	–	+	–	–	
H. aegyptius	+	–	–	–	+	+	–	
H. ducreyi	+	–	–	–		+	–	

200 Gram-negative cocco-bacilli. Sources and transmission of bacteria.

GRAM-NEGATIVE COCCO-BACILLI
IDENTIFYING CHARACTERISTICS

Organism	Gram stain	Culture	Biochemical and other tests
Acinetobacter calcaoaceticus	–ve cocco-bacilli	Grows on blood agar and MacConkey	Oxidase –ve, nitrate –ve
Bordetella pertussis	–ve cocco-bacilli	No growth on blood agar	Mercury-like colonies on CCBA[a] medium, oxidase positive, urea –ve
B. parapertussis	–ve cocco-bacilli	Grows on blood agar	Oxidase positive, urea +ve Culture dependent on X[b] and V[c] factors X V + +
Haemophilus influenzae	–ve cocco-bacilli	} Culture on } heated } blood agar	+ +
H. parainfluenzae	–ve cocco-bacilli		– +
H. aegyptius	–ve cocco-bacilli	Difficult to culture from clinical specimens	+ +
H. ducreyi	–ve cocco-bacilli		+ –

[a]Charcoal cephalexin blood agar. [b]X = hematin. [c]V = NADP.

201 Gram-negative cocco-bacilli. Identifying characteristics.

GRAM-NEGATIVE COCCO-BACILLI INFECTIONS

Organism	Major infection	Less common infection	Vaccine preventable?	Incubation period	Period of infectivity
Pasteurella *P. multocida*	Wound infection following animal bites	Septicemia	No	–	–
Brucella *B. abortus* *B. melitensis*	Brucellosis Brucellosis	– –	– –	5–30 days	Not person-to-person
B. suis	Brucellosis	–	–		

202 Gram-negative cocco-bacilli. Infections.

GRAM-NEGATIVE COCCO-BACILLI SOURCES AND TRANSMISSION OF BACTERIA

Organism	Reservoir			Transmission				Comments
	Man	Animal	Env.	Feco-oral	Droplet	Direct	Nosocomial	
Pasteurella multocida	–	+	–	–	–	+	–	
Brucella abortus	–	+	–	+	+	+	–	Cattle
B. melitensis	–	+	–	+	+	+	–	Sheep, goats
B. suis	–	+	–	+	+	+	–	Pigs

203 Gram-negative cocco-bacilli. Sources and transmission of bacteria.

**GRAM-NEGATIVE COCCO-BACILLI
IDENTIFYING CHARACTERISTICS**

Organism	Gram stain	Culture	Biochemical and other tests	
Pasteurella multocida	–ve cocco-bacilli	Small, non-hemolytic colonies on blood agar	Oxidase +ve, urease –ve	
Brucella abortus	–ve cocco-bacilli	Small, smooth colonies, after 48 h on blood agar Clinical specimen may take up to 4 weeks to grow	Differentiation by dye inhibition tests	
			Thionine	Fuchsin
			+	–
B. melitensis	–ve cocco-bacilli	"	–	–
B. suis	–ve cocco-bacilli	"	–	+
+ = Inhibition.				

204 Gram-negative cocco-bacilli. Identifying characteristics.

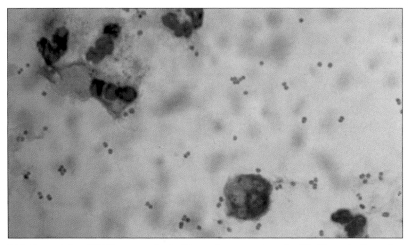

205 Gram stain of CSF from a patient with meningococcal meningitis. The stain shows the Gram-negative diplococci of *Neisseria meningitidis* arranged in pairs and the pink-stained leucocytes. *(Gram stain, ×1000)*

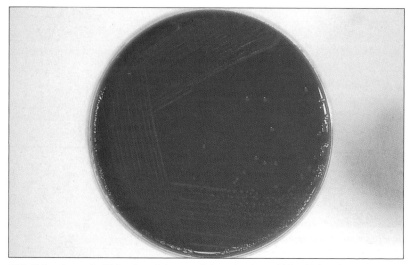

206 Neisseria meningitidis, chocolate agar. Cultured on heated blood ('chocolate') agar, N. meningitidis forms pale gray colonies, which are oxidase positive. *(Heated blood agar, 18 h at 37ºC)*

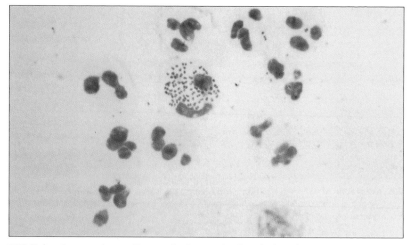

207 Neisseria gonorrhoeae, Gram stain. Gram stain of urethral pus from a patient with gonorrhea. Note that the diplococci occur mostly intracellularly. *(Gram stain, ×1000)*

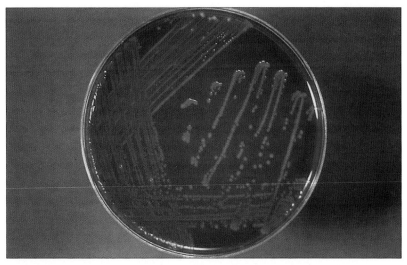

208 Culture of *Neisseria gonorrhoeae*, Modified New York City (MNYC) medium. MNYC is a selective medium for the isolation of *N. gonorrhoeae* from urogenital specimens. *(MNYC agar, 18 h in CO_2 at 37ºC)*

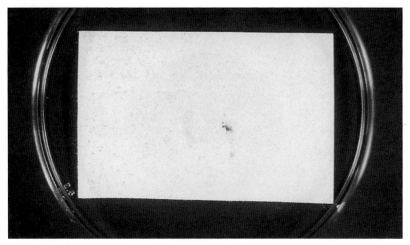

209 *Neisseria gonorrhoeae* oxidase test. *Neisseria* spp are oxidase positive. The isolate is scraped on to a filter paper moistened with oxidase reagent containing phenylene diamine, which is oxidized to purple indophenol. *(Oxidase reagent-soaked paper, read after 30 seconds)*

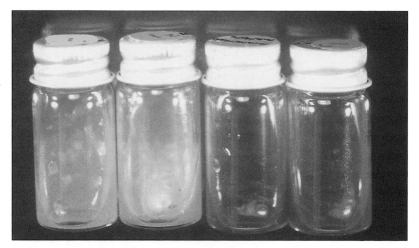

210 Carbohydrate utilization test for *Neisseria*. *Neisseria* spp (in this case *N. meningitidis*) can be distinguished by carbohydrate utilization reactions using glucose, maltose, lactose and sucrose. Acid production is indicated by a yellow color. *(Neisseria sugar medium with phenol red indicator, 18 h at 37ºC)*

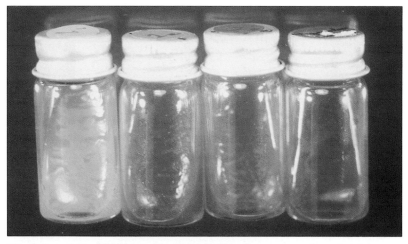

211 Carbohydrate utilization test for *Neisseria*. *Neisseria gonorrhoeae* ferments only glucose. *(Neisseria sugar medium with phenol red indicator, 18 h at 37ºC)*

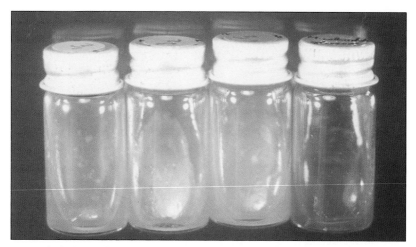

212 Carbohydrate utilization test for _Neisseria_. _Neisseria lactamica_ ferments glucose, maltose and lactose. _(Neisseria sugar medium with phenol red indicator, 18 h at 37ºC)_

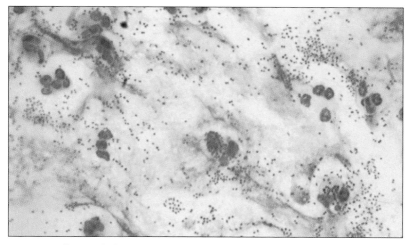

213 _Moraxella catarrhalis_. Gram stain of sputum, showing large Gram-negative cocci. _Moraxella catarrhalis_ is a commensal of the upper respiratory tract but may also cause upper respiratory and other infections. _(Gram stain, ×1000)_

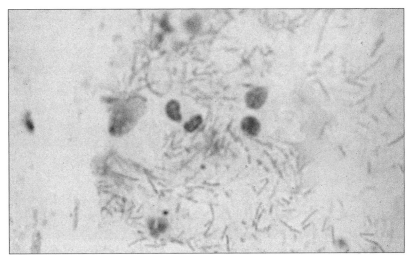

214 *Moraxella lacunata.* Gram stain of eye discharge from patient with conjunctivitis, showing Gram-negative cocco-bacilli, often appearing brick shaped and joined end to end. *(Gram stain, ×1000)*

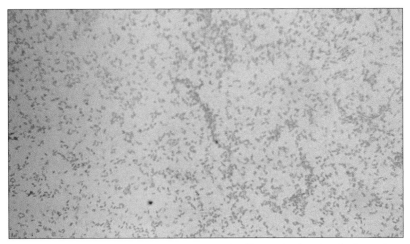

215 *Bordetella pertussis.* The Gram-negative cocco-bacilli occur singly or in pairs. Pertussis (whooping cough) continues to be an important infection of children. Specimens are collected by a per nasal swab and plated on a selective medium such as charcoal cephalexin blood agar. *(Gram stain, ×1000)*

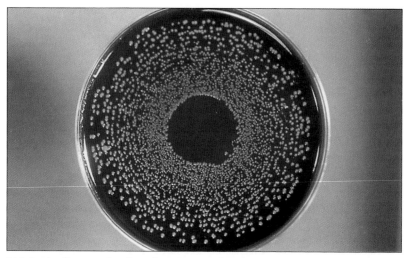

216 *Bordetella pertussis*, **culture from a per nasal swab.** Culture on charcoal cephalexin blood agar (CCBA). After 2–5 days' culture in a moist aerobic atmosphere, *B. pertussis* produces small, shiny, mercury-like colonies. *(CCBA, 5 days at 37°C)*

Clinical specimens are cultured on a selective medium such as charcoal cephalexin blood agar (CCBA) and need to be incubated for 2–3 days. The colonies have a metallic or mercury-like appearance (**216**).

Haemophilus spp

Haemophilus spp include a number of species pathogenic to humans. *Haemophilus influenzae* has both capsulated and non-capsulated strains. Encapsulated strain serotype b is a cause of meningitis and epiglotitis. **217–219** show the Gram-stained appearance of *H. influenzae*. The culture of *Haemophilus* spp requires the growth factors hemin (X) and/or nicotinamide-adenine diphosphate (V). *Haemophilus influenzae* requires both, which are provided by heated blood agar (**220**). The differentiation of *Haemophilus* spp by X and V factor dependence is shown in **221** and **222**. **223** demonstrates the increased growth of *H. influenzae* on blood agar close to a streak of *S. aureus* (satellitism), which provides additional V factor.

Pasteurella spp

Pasteurella multocida is part of the oral flora of dogs and cats, and may cause infection in bite wounds (**224**, **225**).

Brucella spp

Brucellosis in humans may be caused by *Brucella abortus* (from cattle), *B. melitensis* (from sheep and goats) or *B. suis* (from pigs). **226** is a Gram stain of *B. abortus* showing the small, Gram-negative cocco-bacilli.

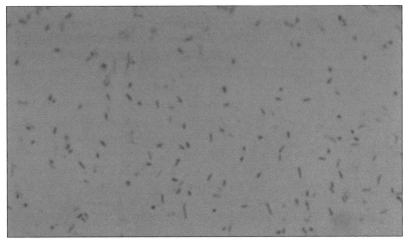

217 *Haemophilus influenzae*. Gram stain from a culture, showing the Gram-negative cocco-bacilli. *(Gram stain, ×1000)*

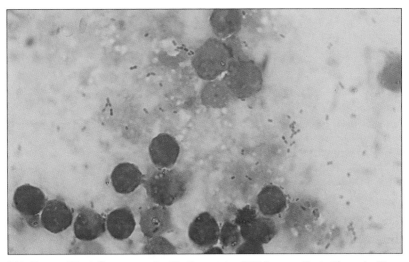

218 *Haemophilus influenzae* meningitis. Gram stain of CSF from a patient with meningitis caused by *H. influenzae*. The Gram-negative cocco-bacilli are sometimes difficult to see among the pink-stained polymorphs. *(Gram stain, ×1000)*

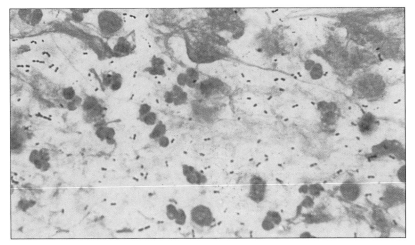

219 *Haemophilus influenzae*. Gram stain of sputum showing *H. influenzae* (Gram-negative cocco-bacilli) and *Streptococcus pneumoniae* (Gram-positive diplococci). *(Gram stain, ×1000)*

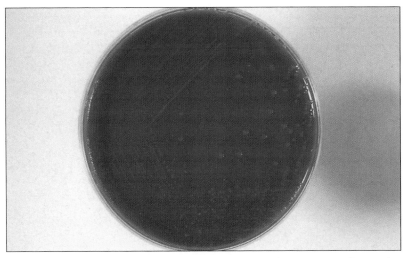

220 *Haemophilus influenzae*, 'chocolate' agar. *Haemophilus influenzae* requires the growth factors hemin (X factor) and nicotinamide adenine dinucleotide (NAD, V factor). V factor is released when blood is heated. The colonies are gray with a mucoid appearance. *(Heated blood agar, 18 h at 37°C)*

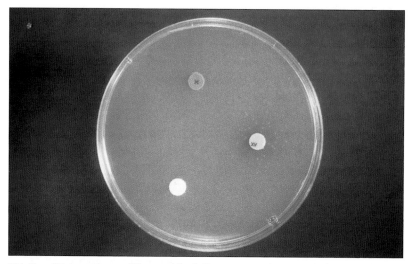

221 X and V dependence of *Haemophilus influenzae*. Growth on nutrient agar with X, V and X+V disks. *Haemophilus influenzae* requires both X and V factors, and only grows around the disk containing X and V. *(Nutrient agar, 18 h at 37°C)*

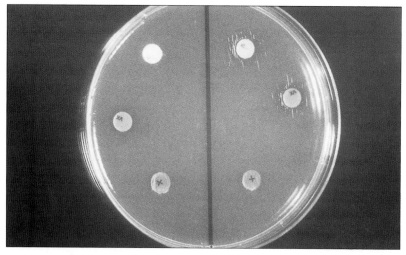

222 *Haemophilus influenzae* and *H. parainfluenzae*. The two halves of the plate are inoculated with *H. influenzae* and *H. parainfluenzae*. *Haemophilus parainfluenzae* requires only V factor and grows round the V and the X+V disks. *(Nutrient agar, 18 h at 37°C)*

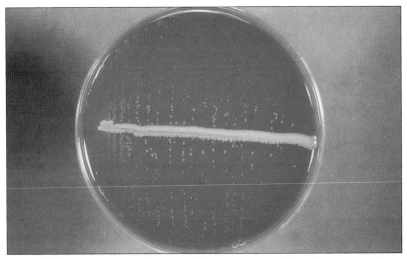

223 Effect of *Staphylococcus aureus* on the growth of *Haemophilus influenzae.* Growth on blood agar showing satellitism adjacent to a streak of *S. aureus. Staphylococcus aureus* produces surplus V factor, increasing the growth of the adjacent *H. influenzae. (Blood agar, 18 h at 37ºC)*

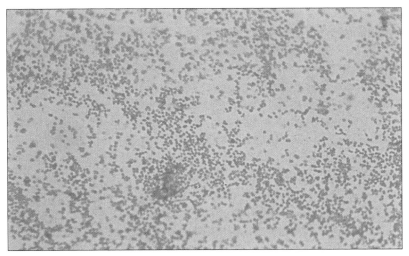

224 *Pasteurella multocida,* Gram stain. *Pasteurella multocida* appears as Gram-negative cocco-bacilli. It is part of the oral flora of dogs and may be a cause of infection in bite wounds. *(Gram stain, ×1000)*

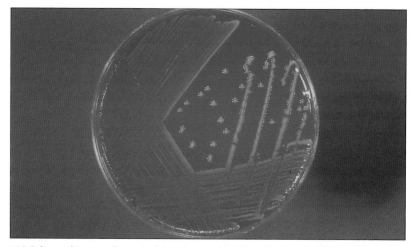

225 Culture of *Pasteurella multocida*. Culture on blood agar showing small, translucent, non-hemolytic colonies with a blue coloration. *Pasteurella multocida* is oxidase positive and does not grow on MacConkey medium. *(Blood agar, 18 h at 37ºC)*

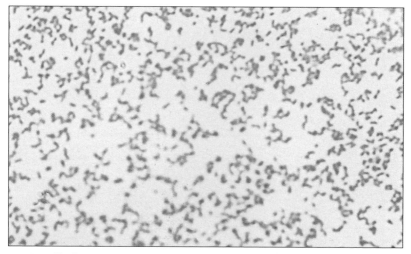

226 *Brucella abortus*. Gram stain, showing Gram-negative cocco-bacilli. The organisms may show bipolar staining and are rarely found in direct smears from uncultured specimens. *(Gram stain, ×1000)*

The different *Brucella* spp may be distinguished by growth inhibition by the dyes thionine and fuchsin (**227**). Contamination of milk by brucella may be demonstrated by the milk ring test (**228**). The rose bengal test is a serological screening test for brucellosis in cattle (**229**).

Vibrios, Campylobacters, *Legionella* and *Garderella*

The characteristics of these bacteria are summarized in **230–232**.

Cholera is caused by the vibrios *V. cholerae* 01 and *V. cholerae* 0139. *Vibrio cholerae* is a comma-shaped, Gram-negative bacillus (**233**). Vibrios can be seen in unstained fecal specimens by dark-field microscopy and grow readily in alkaline peptone-water (**234**). The selective medium thiosulfate, citrate bile salt, sucrose (TCBS) agar is used to isolate *V. cholerae* from feces, giving yellow, oxidase-positive colonies (**235**). Different *V. cholerae* serotypes will grow on TCBS, the confirmation of 01 or 0139 serotype being achieved by

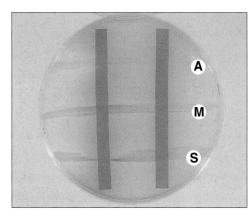

227 Dye inhibition tests for the identification of *Brucella* species. *Brucella* spp may be distinguished by their susceptibility to the dyes basic fuchsin and thionine. Filter papers soaked in the dyes are incorporated in the media and the isolates streaked across them. Fuchsin/thionine: **A** *Brucella abortus* +/–. **M** *Brucella melitensis* +/+. **S** *Brucella suis* –/+. *(Blood agar, 4 days in CO$_2$ at 37°C; + = growth)*

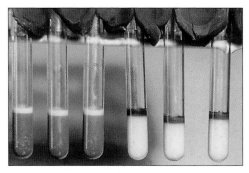

228 Brucella milk ring test. Milk from animals infected with brucellosis may contain brucella agglutinins. Hematoxylin-stained, killed *Brucella* are added to a sample of the milk. A positive test is shown by agglutination and the formation of a blue ring in the sample. *(Incubation for 1 h at 37°C)*

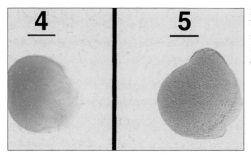

229 Rose bengal test for *Brucella*. The rose bengal test is a serological screening test for *Brucella* antibodies in animals. *(Card agglutination read after 3 min; 5 = positive)*

VIBRIOS AND RELATED SPECIES, LEGIONELLA AND GARDNERELLA INFECTIONS

Organism	Major infection	Less common infection	Vaccine preventable?	Incubation period	Period of infectivity
Vibrio					
V. cholerae	Cholera	–	Yes	2–3 days	May be prolonged
V. parahaemolyticus	Food poisoning		No	12–36 h	Asymptomatic carriage
Aeromonas					
A. hydrophila	Gastroenteritis	Bacteremia in immunocompromised	No	–	–
Plesiomonas					
P. shigelloides	Gastroenteritis	Septicemia	No	–	–
Campylobacter					
C. jejuni	Diarrhea, enterocolitis	Bacteremia	No	1–10 days	Several weeks
Helicobacter					
H. pylori	Gastritis, peptic ulcer	–	No	–	–
Legionella					
L. pneumophila	Legionnaires' disease, fever, cough, myalgia	Pontiac fever	No	2–10 days	Not directly transmitted
Gardnerella					
G. vaginalis	Bacterial vaginosis	–	No	–	–

230 Vibrios and related species, *Legionella* and *Gardnerella*. Infections.

VIBRIOS AND RELATED SPECIES, *LEGIONELLA* AND *GARDNERELLA* SOURCES AND TRANSMISSION OF BACTERIA								
	Reservoir			Transmission				
Organism	**Man**	**Animal**	**Env.**	**Feco-oral**	**Droplet**	**Direct**	**Nosocomial**	**Comments**
Vibrio cholerae	+	–	+	+	–	–	–	Cholera caused by serotypes 01 and 0139
V. para-haemolyticus	–	+	+/–	+	–	–	+	
Aeromonas hydrophila	+	+/–	+	+	–	–	–	
Plesiomonas shigelloides	–	+	+	+	–	–	–	
Campylobacter jejuni	–	+		+		–		
Helicobacter pylori	+				+		+	
Legionella pneumophila	–	–	+	–	–	–	–	
Gardnerella vaginalis	+	–	–	–		+		

231 Vibrios and related species, *Legionella* and *Gardnerella*. Sources and transmission of bacteria.

slide agglutination (**236**). There are two biotypes of *V. cholerae* 01, classical and El-Tor. They may be distinguished by determining sensitivity (classical) or resistance (El-Tor) to polymyxin (**237**). *Vibrio parahaemolyticus* is a cause of food-poisoning and produces green colonies on TCBS (**238**).

Aeromonas hydrophila is a curved, Gram-negative bacillus that is a cause of diarrhea and occasionally septicemia. It grows on blood agar containing ampicillin, producing small hemolytic colonies (**239**). **240** and **241** show *Campylobacter jejuni*, a frequent cause of gastroenteritis. The Gram stain shows delicate 'seagull' shaped, Gram-negative bacilli. *Campylobacter jejuni* is cultured on a selective medium containing vancomycin and colistin, and grows best in micro-aerophillic conditions at 42°C. Other *Campylobacter* spp that are less common causes of diarrheal disease are C. *coli*, C. *lari* and C. *upsaliensis*.

Helicobacter pylori is associated with gastritis and peptic ulcer. It may be demonstrated by the Giemsa staining of gastric biopsies (**242**) or cultured on blood agar (**243**) from a biopsy of gastric mucosa. It is identified by its Gram-stained appearance and possession of a powerful urease.

VIBRIOS AND RELATED SPECIES, *LEGIONELLA* AND *GARDNERELLIA* IDENTIFYING CHARACTERISTICS

Organism	Gram stain	Culture	Biochemical and other tests
Vibrio cholerae	–ve comma-shaped bacilli	Yellow colonies on TCBS[a]	Oxidase +ve. Classical and El-Tor biotypes: distinguished by colistin sensitivity and VP test
V. para-haemolyticus	–ve comma-shaped bacilli	Green colonies on TCBS[a]	Oxidase +ve
Aeromonas hydrophila	–ve vacilli	Beta hemolytic on blood agar	Oxidase +ve, VP +ve
Plesiomonas shigelloides	–ve bacilli	Non-hemolytic on blood agar	Oxidase +ve, VP –ve
Campylobacter jejuni	–ve, thin, S-shaped bacilli	Growth preferred at 43ºC, micro-aerophilic	Inositol fermenter, oxidase +ve
Helicobacter pylori	Curved –ve bacilli	Up to 7 days for growth on chocolate agar	Oxidase +ve
Legionella pneumophila	–ve bacilli	Gray colonies on BCYE[b] agar after 3–4 days	Diagnosis by immunofluorescent test
Gardnerella vaginalis	–ve cocco-bacilli	Gray colonies on selective media in CO_2	'Clue cells' on microscopy

[a]Thiosulfate, citrate, bile salt and sucrose. [b]Buffered charcoal, yeast extract agar.

232 Vibrios and related species, *Legionella* and *Gardnerella*. Identifying characteristics.

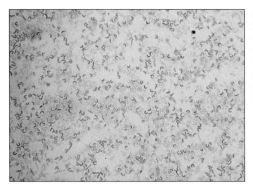

233 *Vibrio cholerae*. Gram stain from alkaline peptone-water culture, showing the Gram-negative, comma-shaped bacilli of *V. cholerae*. Their characteristic appearance can help in the presumptive diagnosis of cholera. *(Gram stain, ×1000)*

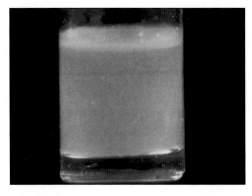

234 Culture of *Vibrio cholerae*, alkaline peptone-water. After 6 h at room temperature, visible growth can be seen at the air–liquid interface. Alkaline peptone-water is a useful transport medium for feces or rectal swabs from suspected cholera cases. *(Alkaline peptone-water, 6 h at room temperature)*

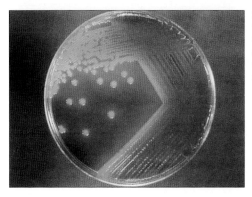

235 *Vibrio cholerae*. Culture on thiosulfate, citrate, bile salt, sucrose (TCBS) agar. *Vibrio cholerae* ferments sucrose and produces yellow colonies. It is oxidase positive. *(TCBS agar, 18 h at 37°C)*

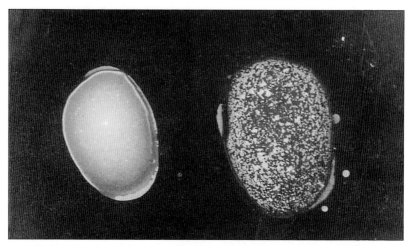

236 *Vibrio cholerae* agglutination. Agglutination of *V. cholerae* serogroup 01 with 01 antiserum by slide agglutination. A dilute suspension of *V. cholerae* from a nutrient agar culture is mixed with a drop of 01 antiserum on the slide and inspected after 30 sec. *(Slide agglutination read after 30 sec)*

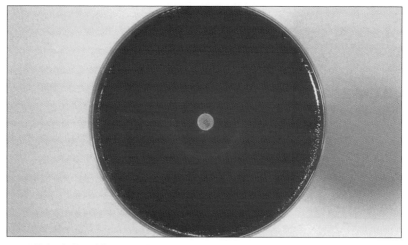

237 *Vibrio cholerae* biotypes. *Vibrio cholerae* 01 is divided into two biotypes: classical and El-Tor. Most cases of cholera now result from the El-Tor biotype. Culture on sensitivity test agar containing a 50 IU polymyxin disk can differentiate El-Tor (resistant) from classical (sensitive) *V. cholerae*. *(Sensitivity test agar, 18 h at 37°C)*

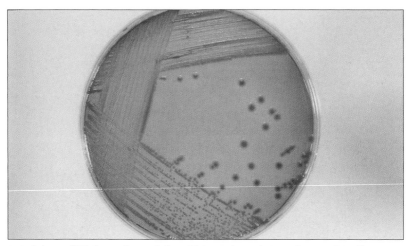

238 Culture of *Vibrio parahaemolyticus.* *Vibrio parahaemolyticus* culture on thiosulfate, citrate, bile salt, sucrose (TCBS) agar showing green (non sucrose-fermenting) colonies. *Vibrio parahaemolyticus* is a cause of food poisoning associated with shellfish and other seafood. *(TCBS agar, 18 h at 37ºC)*

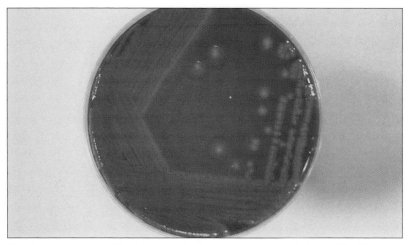

239 *Aeromonas hydrophila.* Culture on blood agar containing 10 μg/ml ampicillin. The small, beta hemolytic colonies are oxidase positive. *(Blood agar, 18 h at 37ºC)*

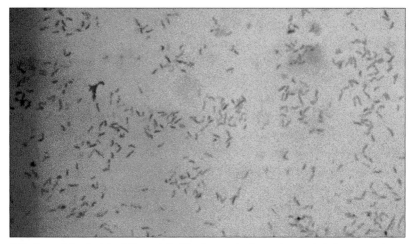

240 *Campylobacter jejuni*, **Gram stain.** The Gram stain shows characteristic Gram-negative, spirally curved bacilli, often described as 'gull wings'. *(Gram stain, ×1000)*

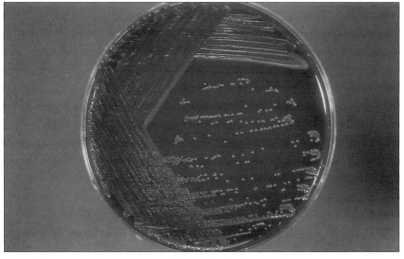

241 Culture of *Campylobacter jejuni*. *Campylobacter jejuni* are micro-aerophilic and grow best at 42ºC. On *Campylobacter*-selective medium, containing antibiotics including vancomycin and polymixin, the colonies are small, gray and droplet-like. *(Campylobacter-selective medium, 48 h, 10% O$_2$ at 43ºC)*

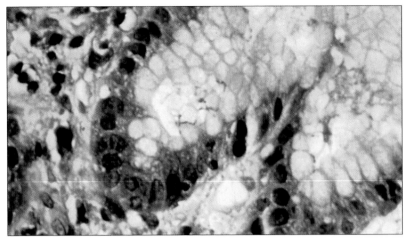

242 *Helicobacter pylori*, **Giemsa stain.** Giemsa stain from a biopsy of gastric mucosa showing *H. pylori* on mucosal cells. *(Giemsa stain, ×1000)*

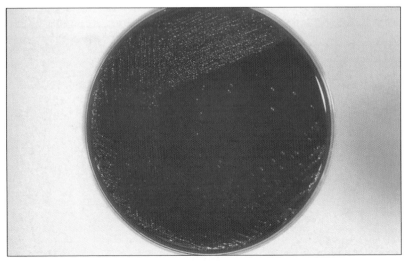

243 *Helicobacter pylori*, **blood agar.** The culture shows pale colonies, which may be grown from gastric biopsy specimens. *(Blood agar, 18 h at 37ºC)*

Legionella pneumophila, the cause of Legionnaire's disease, requires culture for up to 5 days on a selective medium such as buffered charcoal, yeast extract agar (BCYE) (**244**). Specimens may also be investigated directly for *L. pneumophila* by immunofluoresence (**245**).

Gardnerella vaginalis is associated with bacterial vaginosis. Gram staining of a discharge shows epithelial cells surrounded by the pleomorphic Gram-negative bacilli (**246**). **247** shows *G. vaginalis* cultured on a *Gardnerella*-selective agar.

Pseudomonads and other Non-fermentative Gram-negative Bacilli

These are summarized in **248–250**.

Pseudomonads and related species include bacteria that are widely distributed in the environment, some of which are important human pathogens. *Pseudomonas* spp are resistant to many of the commonly available antibiotics. *Pseudomonas aeruginosa* causes a range of infections, including wound infections, urinary tract infections and septicemia. **251** shows a Gram stain of sputum showing the Gram-positive cocci of *S. aureus* and the Gram-negative bacilli of *Ps. aeruginosa. Pseudomonas aeruginosa* is a non-lactose fermenter and is oxidase positive. It often produces a green pigment (pyocyanin) on culture (**252**). Biochemically, *Pseudomonas* spp can be distinguished from Enterobacteriaceae by oxidation–fermentation reactions (**253**).

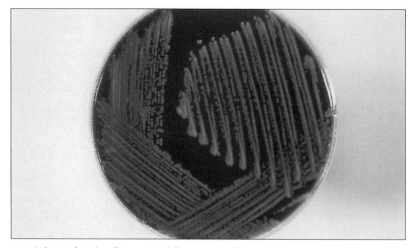

244 Culture of *Legionella pneumophila*. Specimens for *L. pneumophila* are cultured on buffered charcoal, yeast extract (BCYE) medium and incubated in air for up to 2 weeks. Colonies are glistening, gray-white and composed of Gram-negative bacilli. *(BCYE medium, 4 days at 37ºC)*

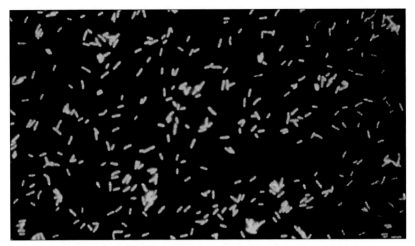

245 Fluorescence microscopy of *Legionella pneumophila*. *Legionella pneumophila* may be detected in respiratory secretions by fluorescein-labeled antibodies using fluorescence microscopy. *(Fluorescence microscopy, ×1000)*

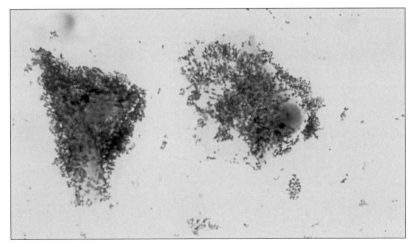

246 *Gardnerella vaginalis*, Gram stain. The Gram stain shows the Gram-negative bacilli of *G. vaginalis* attached to the periphery of epithelial cells, sometimes called 'clue-cells'. *(Gram stain, ×1000)*

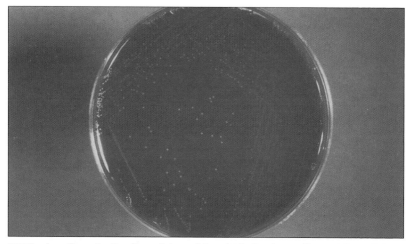

247 *Gardnerella vaginalis* culture. Culture of *G. vaginalis* showing small, gray colonies on *Gardnerella* medium, a Columbia agar base containing gentamicin, nalidixic acid and amphotericin. *(Gardnerella medium, 48 h in CO$_2$ at 37ºC)*

PSEUDOMONADS AND OTHER NON-FERMENTATIVE GRAM-NEGATIVE BACILLI INFECTIONS					
Organism	Major infection	Less common infection	Vaccine preventable?	Incubation period	Period of infectivity
Pseudomonads					
P. aeruginosa	Wound infections, urinary tract, septicemia	Pneumonia	No	–	–
Burkholderia cepacia	Respiratory infections in cystic fibrosis	–	No	–	–
B. pseudomallei	Meliodosis	–	No	Up to several years	Person-to-person unlikely
Stenotrophomonas maltophilia	–	Bacteremia	No	–	–
Eikenella					
E. corrodens	Human bite wounds	Meningitis, endocarditis	No	–	–
Flavobacterium					
F. meningosepticum	Neonatal meningitis	Wound infections	No	–	–

248 Psuedomonads and other non-fermenting, Gram-negative bacilli. Infections.

PSEUDOMONADS AND OTHER NON-FERMENTATIVE GRAM-NEGATIVE BACILLI INFECTIONS (Cont'd)

Organism	Major infection	Less common infection	Vaccine preventable?	Incubation period	Period of infectivity
Kingella *K. kingae*	Arthritis in children	Bacteremia	No	–	–
Dysgonic fermenters DF 3 (*Capnocytophoga canimorsus*)	Animal bites, septicemia		No	–	–

248 Psuedomonads and other non-fermentative, Gram-negative bacilli. Infections

PSEUDOMONADS AND OTHER NON-FERMENTATIVE, GRAM-NEGATIVE BACILLI SOURCES AND TRANSMISSION OF BACTERIA

Organism	Reservoir			Transmission					Comments
	Man	Animal	Env.	Insect	Feco-oral	Droplet	Direct	Nosocomial	
Pseudomonas aeruginosa	+	–	+	–	–	+	+	+	
Burkholderia cepacia	+	–	+	–	–	+	+	+	
Steno-trophomonas maltophilia	–	–	+	–	–	–	+	+	
B. pseudomallei	–	+/–	+	–	–	–	+	–	Saprophytic in soil, occasional human infections in South East Asia
Eikenella corrodens	+	–	–	–	–	–	+	–	
Flavo bacterium meningo-septicum	–	–	+	–	–	–	+	+	
Kingella kingae	+	–	–	–	–	–	+	+	
DF 3	–	+	–	–	–	–	+	–	

249 Pseudomonads and other non-fermentative, Gram-negative bacilli. Sources and transmission of bacteria.

PSEUDOMONADS AND OTHER NON-FERMENTATIVE GRAM-NEGATIVE BACILLI IDENTIFYING CHARACTERISTICS

Organism	Gram stain	Culture	Biochemical and other tests
Pseudomonas aeruginosa	–ve bacilli	Greenish pigment on blood agar	
Burkholderia cepacia	–ve bacilli	Grows on media with colistin	
Stenotrophomonas maltophilia	–ve bacilli	Rough colonies on blood agar	
B. pseudomallei	–ve bacilli, often bipolar	Wrinkled colonies on blood agar	
Eikenella corrodens	–ve bacilli	Pitting colonies on blood agar	
Flavobacterium meningosepticum	Filamentous –ve bacilli	Yellow colonies on blood agar	
Kingella kingae	Short, –ve bacilli	'Fried egg' colonies on blood agar	
DF 3	–ve cocco-bacilli	Nutritionally fastidious Oxidase –ve	All are oxidase +ve except *S. maltophilia*. *Kingella* is an OF-fermenter (glucose); the remainder are non-fermenters

250 Pseudomonads and other non-fermentative, Gram-negative bacilli. Identifying characteristics.

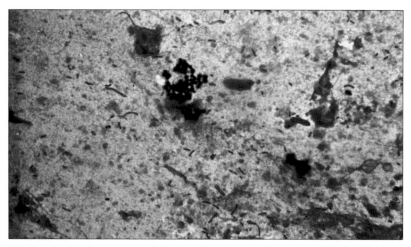

251 Gram stain of sputum containing *Pseudomonas aeruginosa*. Sputum from a patient with cystic fibrosis showing staphylococci and the thin, Gram-negative bacilli of *Ps. aeruginosa*. *(Gram stain, ×1000)*

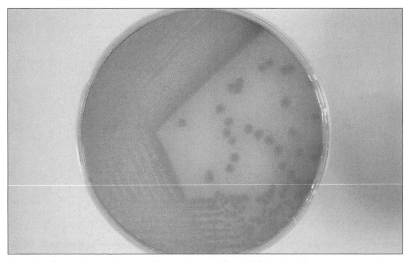

252 *Pseudomonas aeruginosa*. Culture on MacConkey medium. *Pseudomonas aeruginosa* is a non-lactose fermenter and often produces a greenish pyocyanin pigment. It is oxidase positive. *(MacConkey agar, 18 h at 37ºC)*

Burkholderia cenocepacia (formerly *Pseudomonas cepacia*) is an important respiratory pathogen in patients with cystic fibrosis and can be detected by its resistance to colistin (**254**). *Burkholderia pseudomallei* causes the tropical human infection meliodosis (**255–257**).

Eikenella corrodens occurs in human bite wounds. It produces white colonies on blood agar (**258**), which may 'pit' the agar. Flavobacteria include *F. meningosepticum*, a cause of neonatal meningitis, and *F. odoratum*, an occasional pathogen in the immunocompromised. Flavobacteria produce yellow colonies on blood agar (**259**).

■ OBLIGATE ANAEROBIC BACTERIA

The characteristics of anaerobic bacteria are summarized in **260–262**.

Clostridium spp.

Clostridia are spore-forming, Gram-positive cocci including the causative agents of gas gangrene, food poisoning, tetanus, botulism and antibiotic-associated colitis. **263** is a Gram stain from gas gangrene showing the brick-shaped, Gram-positive bacilli of *C. perfringens*. **264** shows the bacilli of *C. tetani* with terminal spores.

Clostridia will grow on blood agar, producing zones of hemolysis (**265, 266**). Clostridia can be distinguished by their reactions in Robinson's cooked

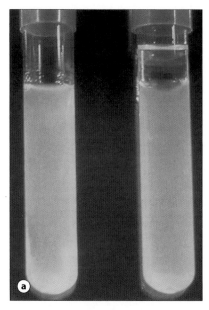

253 Oxidation–fermentation reactions. The test organism is inoculated into two tubes of a tryptone agar medium containing glucose and the indicator bromothymol blue. The medium in one tube is sealed with a layer of liquid paraffin to exclude oxygen. The tubes are incubated for up to 7–14 days; acid production is indicated by a yellow color. Bacteria that both oxidize and ferment glucose produce acid in both tubes, but oxidizers that do not ferment glucose produce acid in only the unsealed tube. **a** *Escherichia coli*. Oxidation plus fermentation. **b** *Pseudomonas aeruginosa*. Acid is produced only in the oxidative tube (left), showing that *Ps. aeruginosa* is a non-fermenter. *(Trypton agar, 7 days at 37ºC)*

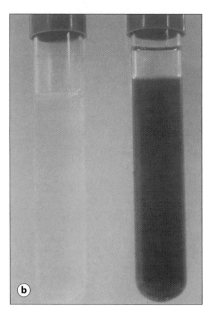

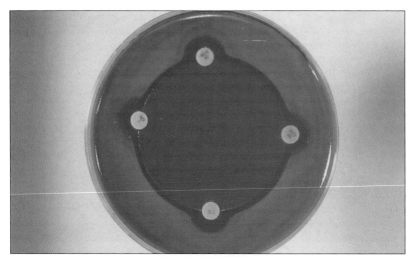

254 *Burkholderia cepacia.* *Burkholderia cepacia* (formerly *Pseudomonas cepacia*) is an increasingly important respiratory pathogen in cystic fibrosis patients. Most strains are multiply antimicrobial resistant. *Burkholderia cepacia* is inoculated centrally. A sensitive control is inoculated peripherally. *(Sensitivity test agar, 18 h at 37°C)*

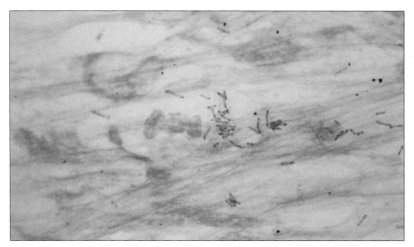

255 *Burkholderia pseudomallei.* Gram stain of *B. pseudomallei* in sputum. The organism is pleomorphic and may show bipolar staining. *(Gram stain, ×1000)*

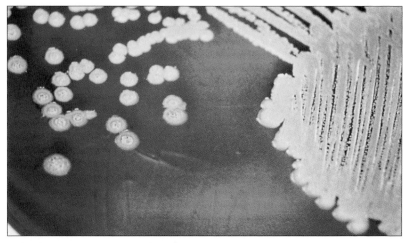

256 Burkholderia pseudomallei, blood agar. Culture after 72 h showing characteristic dry, wrinkled colonies. The cultures have a 'truffle' like odor. *(Blood agar, 72 h at 37ºC)*

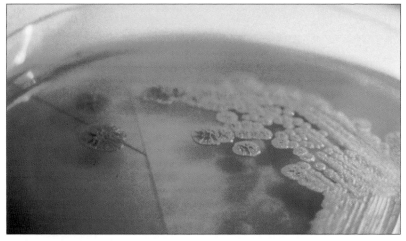

257 Burkholderia pseudomallei, Ashdown's medium. The medium is selective, containing crystal violet and gentamicin. The wrinkled morphology is enhanced by glycerol in the medium. *(Ashdown's medium, 72 h at 37ºC)*

258 *Eikenella corrodens.* Culture on blood agar showing white colonies. When the colonies are scraped from the agar, the agar is often pitted. *(Blood agar, 18 h at 37°C)*

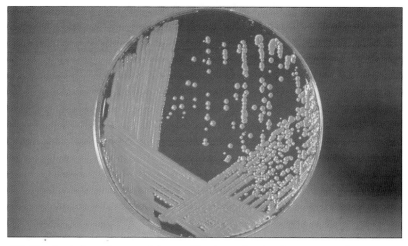

259 *Flavobacterium odoratum.* Culture on blood agar showing characteristic yellow colonies. Flavobacteria are widely disseminated in the environment and are occasional pathogens. *Flavobacterium meningosepticum* is a cause of neonatal meningitis. *(Blood agar, 18 h at 37°C)*

OBLIGATE ANAEROBIC BACTERIA INFECTIONS

Organism	Major infection	Less common infection	Vaccine preventable?	Incubation period	Period of infectivity
Gram-positive					
Clostridium					
C. tetani	Tetanus		Yes	3–21 days	
C. perfringens (C. welchii)	Gas gangrene, food poisoning, wound infections	Puerperal sepsis, pig bel	No	6–24 h 12–36 h	
C. botulinum	Botulism, infant botulism		No (antitoxin available)	2–3 days	
C. difficile	Antibiotic-associated colitis	–	No	–	Up to 4 weeks
Propronibacterium					
P. acnes	Prosthetic device infections	Osteomyelitis, endocarditis	No	–	–
Gram-negative					
Bacteroidaceae					
B. fragilis	Intra-abdominal sepsis, intracerebral abscess	Pneumonia	No	–	–
B. melaninogenicus (Prevotella melaninogenicus)	Abdominal wound		No	–	–
Fusobacterium					
F. nucleatum	Vincent's angina	Tropical ulcer	No	–	–
F. necrophorum	Head/neck infections	Necrobacillosis	No	–	–

260 Obligate anaerobic bacteria. Infections.

ANAEROBIC BACTERIA SOURCES AND TRANSMISSION OF BACTERIA								
	Reservoir			Transmission				
Organism	Man	Animal	Env.	Feco-oral	Droplet	Direct	Nosocomial	Comments
Clostridium tetani	–	+	+	–	–	+	–	
C. perfringens	–	+	+	+	–	–	–	
C. botulinum	–	+	+	+	–	–	–	
C. difficile	+	–	+/–	+	–	+/–	+	Antibiotic-associated diarrhea
Propionibacterium acnes	+	–	+/–	–	–	+	+	
Bacteroides fragilis	+	–	–	–	–	+	+	
B. melanino-genicus	+	–	–	–	–	+	+	
Fusobacterium nucleatum	+	–	–	–	–	+	–	
F. necrophorum	+	–	–	–	–	+	–	

261 Anaerobic bacteria. Sources and transmission of bacteria.

meat medium (**267**), on lactose, egg yolk, milk agar (**268**) and by the Nagler reaction (**269**). *Clostridium difficile* is associated with antibiotic-associated colitis. On cycloserine-cefoxitin, fructose agar (CCFA), it produces ground-glass colonies (**270, 271**). The production of C. *difficile* toxin can be demonstrated by tissue culture cytotoxicity (**272**) or enzyme-linked immunosorbent assay (ELISA).

Anaerobic Gram-negative Bacilli

Bacteroides fragilis is frequently isolated from abdominal abscesses (**273**). *Bacteroides* species can be distinguished by their antimicrobial sensitivity patterns (**274**) and by the volatile fatty acids detected on gas liquid chromatography (**275**). *Bacteroides melaninogenicus* (now *Prevotella melaninogenicus*) produces characteristic brown-black colonies on blood agar (**276**).

Fusobacterium spp are a cause of chronic infections including Vincent's angina, an infection of the jaw in which the spirochaete *Borrelia vincenti* is also involved together with *F. nucleatum*, which are slender, Gram-negative rods, often with pointed ends (**277**). *Fusobacterium necrophorum* is also a cause of infections in the head and neck, and can, with severe infections, lead to septicemia (**278, 279**).

ANAEROBIC BACTERIA
IDENTIFYING CHARACTERISTICS

Organism	Gram stain	Culture	Biochemical and other tests Culture on lactose, egg yolk, milk agar			
			Lecithinase	Lipase	Lactose	Proteinase
Clostridium tetani	Broad +ve bacilli, spores rarely seen	Film of growth on blood agar	–	–	–	–
C. perfringens	+ve bacilli	Beta hemolytic on blood agar	+	–	+	–
C. botulinum	+ve bacilli with oval subterminal spores	Large semi-transparent colonies on blood agar	–	+	–	+
C. difficile	+ve bacilli	'Ground glass' colonies on CCFA[a] agar				
			Antibiotic tests	Col.	Vanc.	Kan.[b]
Bacteroides fragilis	Pleomorphic –ve bacilli	Gray, non-hemolytic colonies on blood agar		R	R	R
B. melaninogenicus	–ve bacilli	Brown-black hemolytic colonies on blood agar		S	R	R
Fusobacterium nucleatum	Fusiform –ve bacilli, pointed ends	Bread crumb-like colonies on blood agar		S	R	S
F. necrophorum	Fusiform –ve bacilli, rounded ends	Pale colonies on blood agar		S	R	S

[a]Cycloserine, cefoxitin, fructose agar. [b]Colistin, vancomycin, kanamycin. S = sensitive. R = resistant.

262 Anaerobic bacteria. Identifying characteristics.

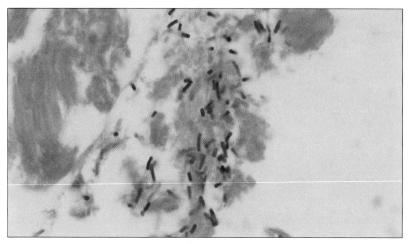

263 *Clostridium perfringens* (*C. welchii*). Gram stain of pus from gas gangrene showing thick, brick-shaped, Gram-positive bacilli. *(Gram stain, ×1000)*

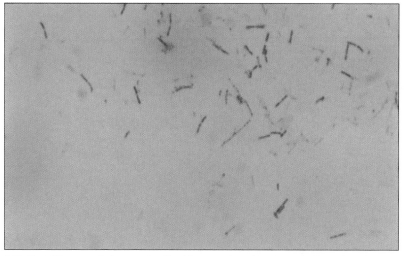

264 *Clostridium tetani*, Gram stain. *Clostridium tetani* are thin, Gram-positive rods with terminal spores. The centers of the spores do not stain. *(Gram stain, ×1000)*

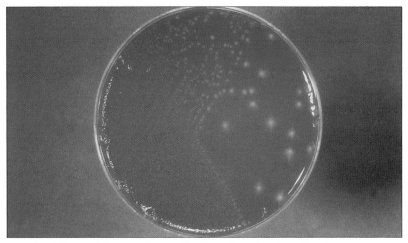

265 *Clostridium perfringens*. Culture on blood agar shows beta hemolysis. Some strains produce a double zone of hemolysis. *(Blood agar, 48 h anaerobically at 37ºC)*

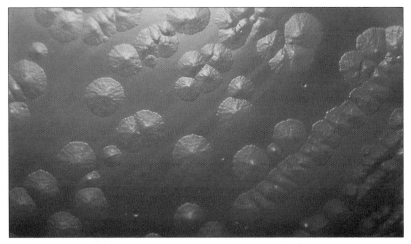

266 *Clostridium perfringens*, blood agar. The colonies show a halo of double hemolysis owing to the different toxins present. *(Blood agar, 48h anaerobically at 37ºC)*

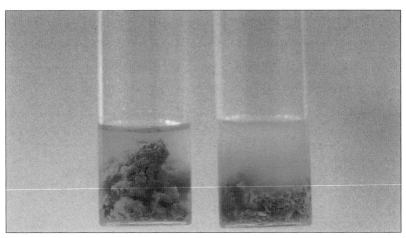

267 *Clostridium perfringens*, **Robertson's cooked meat medium.** Growth in Robertson's cooked meat medium (left) showing saccharolytic (reddening) and slight proteolytic (blackening) reactions. Gas is also produced. Right, uninoculated. *(Cooked meat medium, 24 h at 37ºC)*

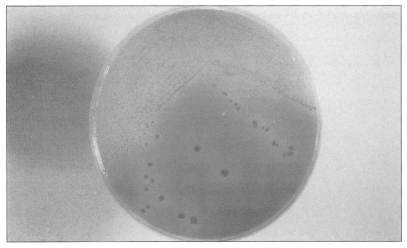

268 *Clostridium perfringens*, **lactose, egg yolk, milk agar.** On lactose, egg yolk, milk agar, *C. perfringens* produces pink colonies as a result of lactose fermentation, surrounded by a zone of opacity owing to the breakdown of lecithin. *(Lactose, egg yolk, milk agar, 48 h anaerobically at 37ºC)*

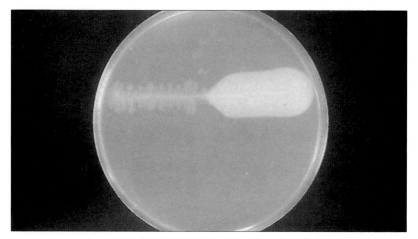

269 Nagler reaction. The Nagler plate contains an egg yolk medium, half of the plate being covered with *C. perfringens* antitoxin. Organisms are streaked across the plate so that inoculum passes from the antitoxin-free half of the plate to the antitoxin-covered part. After overnight anaerobic incubation, a positive result is shown by opacity in the medium surrounding the inoculum on the non-antitoxin half of the plate. Right side, no antitoxin. *(Nagler plate, 18 h anaerobically at 37ºC)*

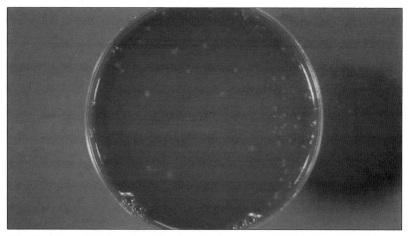

270 *Clostridium difficile*, cycloserine-cefoxitin, fructose agar (CCFA). *Clostridium difficile* is associated with pseudomembranous colitis. On CCFA, the colonies are a shiny, gray color. *(CCFA, 48 h anaerobically at 37ºC)*

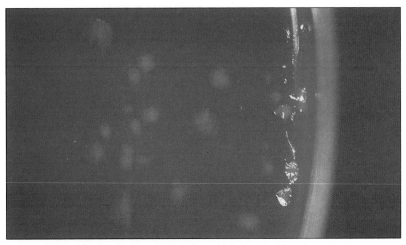

271 *Clostridium difficile*, **charcoal cephalexin blood agar, close-up of colonies.** The 'metallic' shiny appearance of the colonies is demonstrated. *(CCBA, 48 h, anaerobically at 37°C)*

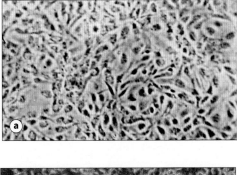

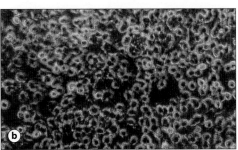

272 Tissue culture showing action of *Clostridium difficile* **toxin.** Colitis and diarrhea are caused by toxin-producing strains of *C. difficile*. Toxin may be demonstrated by its effect on Vero cells after overnight incubation (**b**). **a** Uninoculated. *(Vero cells, 18 h at 37°C)*

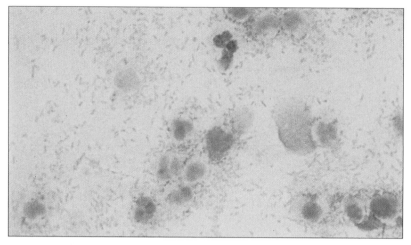

273 *Bacteroides fragilis*, Gram stain. *Bacteroides fragilis* are small, Gram-negative bacilli associated with intra-abdominal abscesses. *(Gram stain, ×1000)*

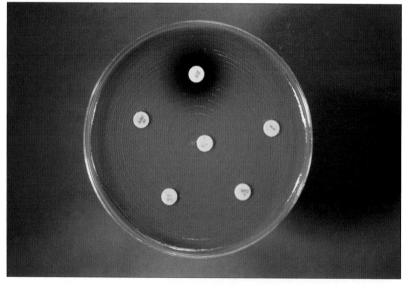

274 Identification of *Bacteroides* spp by antimicrobial sensitivity. Antimicrobial disc sensitivity can aid the identification of *Bacteroides* spp. *Bacteroides fragilis* is resistant to colistin, penicillin, kanamycin and vancomycin, and sensitive to erythromycin and rifampicin. *(DST agar with 5% lysed blood, 48 h anaerobically at 37ºC)*

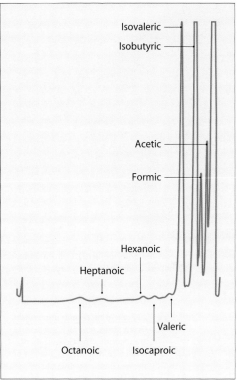

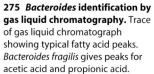

275 *Bacteroides* identification by gas liquid chromatography. Trace of gas liquid chromatograph showing typical fatty acid peaks. *Bacteroides fragilis* gives peaks for acetic acid and propionic acid.

(Labels on chromatograph): Isovaleric, Isobutyric, Acetic, Formic, Hexanoic, Heptanoic, Valeric, Octanoic, Isocaproic

■ **UNCLASSIFIED BACTERIA**

A number of bacteria, including an increasing number of newly described pathogens, do not fall neatly within the standard classification. The characteristics of some of these are summarized in **280–282**. Many of them are difficult to cultivate or are relatively inert biochemically. *Bartonella bacilliformis* is a Gram-negative, coccoid bacterium that is the cause of bartonellosis (Oroya fever), a febrile or chronic cutaneous disease restricted to parts of the Andean region of South America. It may be demonstrated by Giemsia staining of the blood of infected patients (**283**). *Bartonella henselae* has recently been described as the cause of cat scratch fever and bacillary angiomatosis, and is a Gram-negative bacillus (**284**).

■ **MYCOBACTERIA**

Mycobacteria, summarized in **285–287**, include the important pathogens of tuberculosis and leprosy, as well as a large number of environmental strains that are opportunistic pathogens.

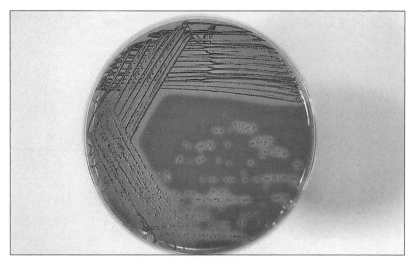

276 *Prevotella melaninogenicus* (formerly *Bacteroides melaninogenicus*). Culture on blood agar showing brown-black colonies after 5 days' incubation. *(Blood agar, 5 days anaerobically at 37°C)*

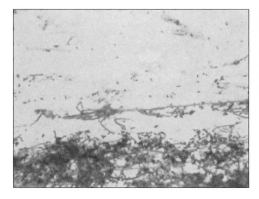

277 *Fusobacterium nucleatum*, Gram stain. Not all fusobacteria are fusiform. The Gram stain of *F. nucleatum* from a jaw infection shows Gram-negative bacilli, some with slender ends. *(Gram stain, ×1000)*

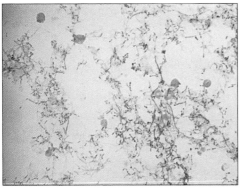

278 *Fusobacterium necrophorum.* Gram stain from a blood culture of a patient with *F. necrophorum* septicemia originating from mastoiditis. *(Gram stain, ×1000)*

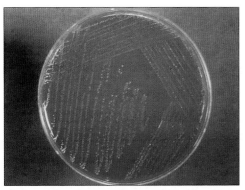

279 *Fusobacterium necrophorum,* **blood agar.** Culture of *F. necrophorum* on blood agar showing small, pale colonies. *(Blood agar, 48 h anaerobically at 37ºC)*

'UNCLASSIFIED' BACTERIA INFECTIONS

Organism	Major infection	Less common infection	Vaccine preventable?	Incubation period
Spirillum minus	Rat-bite fever	–	–	1–3 months
Klebsiella granulomatis	Granuloma inguinale (donovanosis)	–	–	–
Bartonella henselae	Bacillary angiomatosis, cat scratch fever	–	–	–
B. bacilliformis	Oroya fever, verruga peruana	–	–	2 weeks – 4 months
Streptobacillus moniliformis	Rat-bite fever, Haverhill fever	–	–	3–10 days

280 'Unclassified' bacteria. Infections.

'UNCLASSIFIED' BACTERIA
SOURCES AND TRANSMISSION OF BACTERIA

Organism	Reservoir			Transmission					Comments
	Man	Animal	Env.	Insect	Feco-oral	Droplet	Direct	Nosocomial	
Spirillum minus	–	+ Rats		–	–	–	–	–	
Klebsiella granulomatis	+	–	–	–	–	–	+	–	Sexual transmission
Bartonella henselae	–	+	–	–	–	–	+	–	
B. bacilliformis	+	–	–	+ Sandfly	–	–	–	–	Limited to Andean region of Peru and Ecuador
Streptobacillus moniliformis[a]	–	+	+	–	+	±	–	–	

[a]Infection by bite or from contaminated water or milk.

281 'Unclassified' bacteria. Sources and transmission of bacteria.

'UNCLASSIFIED' BACTERIA
IDENTIFYING CHARACTERISTICS

Organism	Gram stain	Culture	Biochemical and other tests
Spirillum minus	Thick, spiral, –ve bacilli	Not cultured in vitro	
Klebsiella granulomatis	–ve cocco-bacilli	Difficult to culture using egg yolk-based medium	
Bartonella henselae	–ve bacilli		
B. bacilliformis	–ve cocco-bacilli	White colonies on blood agar after 7–14 days	Biochemically inert Diagnosis usually by Giemsa stain from blood film
Stretobacillus moniliformis	Pleomorphic -ve cocco-bacilli	Non-hemolytic colonies on blood agar	Indole, oxidase, catalase, nitrate –ve

282 'Unclassified' bacteria. Identifying characteristics.

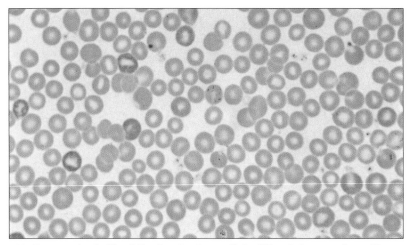

283 Giemsa stain of a blood film showing *Bartonella bacilliformis* from a patient with Oroya fever. The film shows the intracellular cocco-bacilli staining a deep purple. *Bartonella* multiplies in the red cells, causing their destruction and a subsequent anemia. *(Giemsa stain, ×1000)*

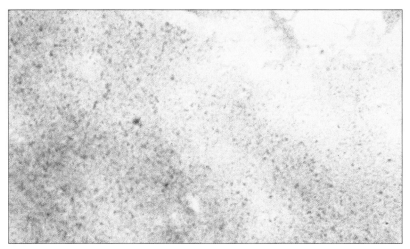

284 *Bartonella henselae*, Gram stain. Showing Gram-negative cocco-bacilli. *Bartonella henselae* is a cause of cat scratch disease and is associated with bacillary angiomatosis. *(Gram stain, ×1000)*

MYCOBACTERIA INFECTIONS					
Organism	Major infection	Less common infection	Vaccine preventable?	Incubation period	Period of infectivity
Mycobacterium tuberculosis	Tuberculosis	–	+/–	4–12 weeks	Indefinite in untreated pulmonary infection
M. bovis	Tuberculosis	–	+/–	4–12 weeks	–
M. ulcerans	Buruli ulcer	–	–		–
M. kansasii	Pulmonary disease	–	–		–
M. marinum	'Fish tank' ulcer	–	–		–
M. scrofulaceum	Cervical lymph-adenopathy	–	–		–
M. malmoense	Cervical lymph-adenopathy	–	–		–
M. avium-intracellulare	Disseminated Infection in immuno-compromised	–	–		–
M. chelonei	Occasional skin infections following minor trauma	–	–		–
M. gordonae	" "	–	–		–
M. xenopi	" "	–	–		–
M. fortuitum	Abscesses	–	–		–
M. leprae	Leprosy	–	+ BCG	4–8 years	Indefinite if not treated

285 Mycobacteria. Infections.

Mycobacteria are stained by the Ziehl– Neelsen method, showing pink, acid-fast bacilli (**288**). Auramine phenol staining may also be used (**289**).

Mycobacteria have exacting nutritional requirements, and will not grow on ordinary media. Löwenstein–Jensen (LJ) medium has ingredients including eggs, glycerol and malachite green. Most mycobacteria are slow growing, taking 4–12 weeks to produce visible colonies. **290** shows *M. tuberculosis* after 6 weeks' culture on LJ medium, with a typical 'breadcrumb'-like appearance. *Mycobacterium bovis* grows better on LJ slopes containing pyruvate rather than glycerol (**291**). **292** and **293** show the 'atypical' mycobacteria, *M. kansasii* and *M. avium-intracellulare*, grown on LJ slopes.

Mycobacteria can be distinguished by the effect of temperature on growth, the production of pigment and the rate of growth. **294** shows mycobacteria with narrow and wide temperature growth ranges.

MYCOBACTERIA SOURCES AND TRANSMISSION OF BACTERIA								
	Reservoir			Transmission				
Organism	Man	Animal	Env.	Feco-oral	Droplet	Direct	Nosocomial	Comments
Mycobacterium tuberculosis	+	–	–	–	+	–	+	
M. bovis		+	–	+	+/–			
M. ulcerans			+			+		
M. kansasii	+		+		+			
M. marinum			+			+		
M. scrofulaceum			+	(+)	+	+		
M. malmoense			+			+		
M. avium-intracellulare	+	+			+			
M. chelonei			+			+		
M. gordonae			+			+		
M. xenopi			+			+		
M. fortuitum			+			+		
M. leprae	+	–	–	–	(+)	+	–	

286 Mycobacteria. Sources and transmission of bacteria.

GROWTH CHARACTERISTICS OF *MYCOBACTERIA*								
	Rate	Temperature				Pigment production		
		25°C	32°C	36°C	44°C	N*	P*	S*
Mycobacterium tuberculosis	S	–	+	+	–	+	–	–
M. bovis	S	–	(+)	+	–	+	–	–
M. ulcerans	S	–	+	–	–	+	–	–
M. kansasii	S	+	+	+	–	–	+	–
M. marinum	S	+	+	±	–	–	+	–
M. scrofulaceum	S	+	+	+	–	–	–	+
M. malmoense	S	+	+	+	+	+	–	–
M. avium-intracellulare	S	+	+	+	+	+	–	+
M. chelonae	R	+	+	+	–	+	–	–
M. gordonae	S	+	+	+	–	–	–	+
M. xenopi	S	–	–	+	+	–	–	+
M. fortuitum	R	+	+	+	–	+	–	–
M. leprae	S(a)							

N* = non-chromogen. P* = photochromogen. S* = scotochromogen. S = slow growth. R = rapid growth. S(a) = not cultivated on artificial media.

287 Growth characteristics of *mycobacteria*.

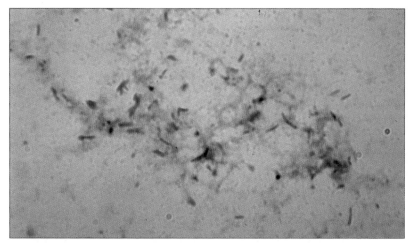

288 *Mycobacterium tuberculosis.* Ziehl–Neelsen staining of sputum from a patient with tuberculosis showing pink, acid-fast bacilli against a blue background of pus cells. *(Ziehl–Neelsen stain, ×1000)*

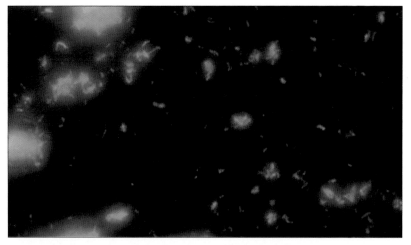

289 *Mycobacterium tuberculosis,* **auramine phenol fluorochrome.** Auramine is a fluorochrome, a dye that fluoresces when illuminated by UV light. Tubercle bacilli fluoresce a white-yellow color. *(Fluorochrome stain, ×1000)*

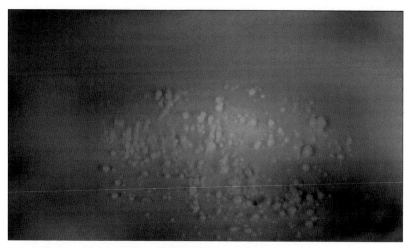

290 *Mycobacterium tuberculosis*, **Löwenstein–Jensen (LJ) medium.** Culture on LJ medium after 6 weeks. The mycobacteria produce creamy, breadcrumb-like colonies. *(LJ medium, 6 weeks at 37ºC)*

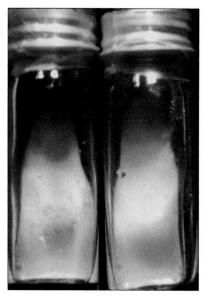

291 *Mycobacterium bovis*,
Löwenstein–Jensen (LJ) medium. Culture on LJ medium containing glycerol (right) and pyruvate (left). Growth of *M. bovis* is better on the pyruvate slope. *(LJ medium, 6 weeks at 37ºC)*

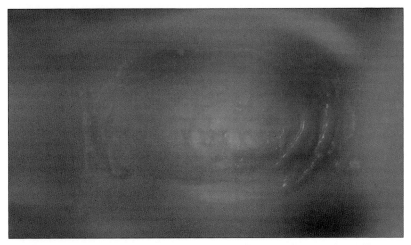

292 *Mycobacterium kansasii*, **Löwenstein–Jensen medium.** *Mycobacterium kansasii* is an opportunistic *Mycobacterium* and is an occasional cause of a tuberculosis-like pulmonary infection. *Mycobacterium kansasii* is a photochromogen. *(LJ medium, 6 weeks at 37ºC)*

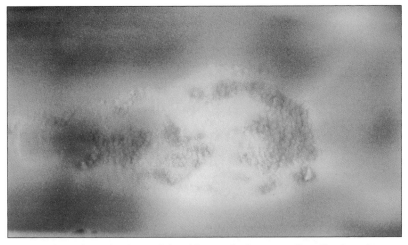

293 *Mycobacterium avium intracellulare*, **Löwenstein–Jensen medium.** *Mycobacterium avium intracellulare* is a potential pathogen in the immunocompromised and is particularly associated with HIV infection. *(LJ medium, 6 weeks at 37ºC)*

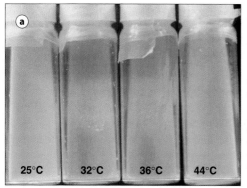

294 Effect of temperature on growth of mycobacteria. Different mycobacteria have different ranges of temperature for growth. The Löwenstein–Jensen slopes have been incubated at 25°C, 32°C, 36°C and 44°C. *(LJ medium, temperatures as indicated).* **a** *Mycobacterium tuberculosis*, growth at 32°C and 36°C. **b** *Mycobacterium kansasii*, growth at 25°C, 32°C and 36°C. **c** *Mycobacterium malmoense*, growth at 25°C, 32°C, 36°C and 44°C.

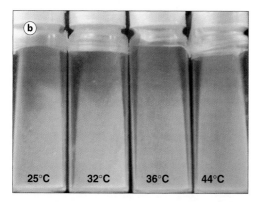

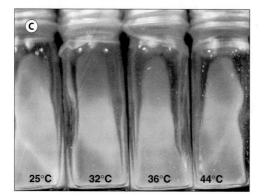

Mycobacteria may be non-pigmented (non-chromogens), produce pigment only in light (photochromogens) or produce pigment in both dark and light (scotochromogens). These are shown in **295**. **296** shows the growth after 10 days of a slow grower, *M. tuberculosis*, and a rapid grower, *M. fortuitum*. **297** shows a Ziehl–Neelsen stain of *M. leprae* from a slit skin smear.

■ MYCOPLASMAS, SPIROCHAETES AND RICKETTSIAE

These microorganisms are summarized in **298–300**, **302–304** and **309**.

Mycoplasmas and ureaplasmas cannot be detected directly in stained specimens. They are slow growing and produce small colonies after several days' incubation (**301**). *Treponema pallidum*, the cause of syphilis, may be demonstrated as tightly wound spirochaetes using dark-field microscopy (**305**). Serological tests are generally used in the investigation of syphilis. Both treponomal specific antibodies, and auto-antibodies (cardiolipin) from tissue damage are produced. The rapid plasma reagin test (**306**) is an example of a cardiolipin test.

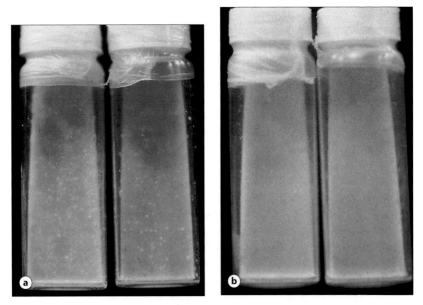

295 Effect of light on mycobacteria. Mycobacteria that produce no pigment are non-chromogens. Those which produce pigment only in the light are photochromogens. Those producing pigment in both light and dark are scotochromogens. In the figures, the left-hand slope was grown in the dark and the right-hand slope in the light. (*Löwenstein–Jensen medium at 37ºC*) **a** *Mycobacterium kansasii*, photochromogen. **b** *Mycobacterium gordonae*, scotochromogen.

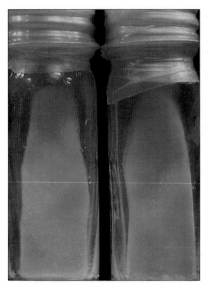

296 Rate of growth of mycobacteria.
Mycobacteria may be divided into rapid and slow growers. Rapid growers will produce colonies in 3–4 days. Most mycobacteria require a minimum of 3–4 weeks before colonies are visible. The slopes have been incubated for 7 days. Right, *Mycobacterium tuberculosis*, no growth. Left, *Mycobacterium fortuitum*, a rapid grower. *(Löwenstein–Jensen medium at 37ºC)*

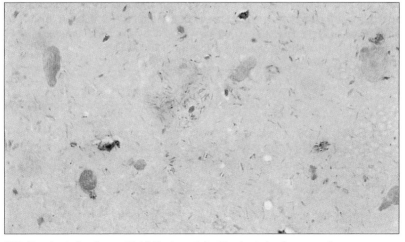

297 *Mycobacterium leprae*, Ziehl–Neelsen stain. *Mycobacterium leprae* may be demonstrated by the staining of slit skin smears with a modified Ziehl–Neelsen stain. It is only weakly acid fast and a 1%, instead of 3%, acid–alcohol solution is used for decolorization. *Mycobacterium leprae* appears as thin, pink bacilli, often within macrophage cells. *(Ziehl–Neelsen stain, ×1000)*

MYCOPLASMA AND *UREAPLASMA* INFECTIONS					
Organism	Major infection	Less common infection	Vaccine preventable?	Incubation period	Period of infectivity
Mycoplasma pneumoniae	Pneumonia, tracheobronchitis	Myocarditis	–	6–21 days	Up to 14 days
M. hominis	Urethritis, postpartum infection pelvic inflammatory disease	Wound infection, neonatal meningitis	–	–	–
Ureaplasma urealyticum	Urethritis	–	–	–	–

298 *Mycoplasma* and *Ureaplasma*. Infections.

MYCOPLASMA AND *UREAPLASMA* SOURCES AND TRANSMISSION OF BACTERIA								
	Reservoir			Transmission				
Organism	Man	Animal	Env.	Feco-oral	Droplet	Direct	Nosocomial	Comments
Mycoplasma pneumoniae	+	–	–	–	+	–	–	
M. hominis	+	–	–	–	–	+	–	
Ureaplasma urealyticum	+	–	–	–	–	+	–	

299 *Mycoplasma* and *Ureaplasma*. Sources and transmission of bacteria.

MYCOPLASMA AND *UREAPLASMA* IDENTIFYING CHARACTERISTICS			
Organism	Microscopy	Culture	Other tests for identification
Mycoplasma pneumoniae	Small, pleomorphic non-motile organisms cannot be detected in stained specimens	Enriched media required Small colonies with 'fried egg' appearance after several days	Serological diagnosis by complement fixation test and ELISA
M. hominis *Ureaplasma urealyticum*			

300 *Mycoplasma* and *Ureaplasma*. Identifying characteristics.

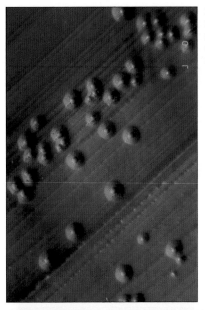

301 Culture of *Mycoplasma hominis*. Close-up of colonies, showing the 'fried-egg' appearance, on mycoplasma enrichment ('pleuropneumonia-like organisms', PPLO) medium. *(PPLO medium, 5 days at 37°C)*

SPIROCHAETES INFECTIONS					
Organism	Major infection	Less common infection	Vaccine preventable?	Incubation period	Period of infectivity
Treponema					
T. pallidum	Syphilis	–	–	1–6 weeks	2–4 years if not treated
T. pertenue	Yaws	–	–	2 weeks – 3 months	Several years if not treated
T. carateum	Pinta	–	–	2–3 weeks	Several years if not treated
Leptospira					
L. interrogans	Leptospirosis (Weil's disease)	–	–	4–20 days	Person-to-person transmission rare
Borrelia					
B. vincenti	Vincent's angina	Tropical ulcer	–	–	–
B. recurrentis	Louse-borne relapsing fever	–	–	5–15 days	–
B. duttoni	Tick-borne relapsing fever	–	–	5–15 days	–
B. burgdorferi	Lyme disease	–	–	3–30 days	–

302 Spirochaetes. Infections.

SPIROCHAETES
SOURCES AND TRANSMISSION OF BACTERIA

Organism	Reservoir			Transmission					Comments
	Man	Animal	Env.	Insect	Feco-oral	Droplet	Direct	Nosocomial	
Treponema pallidum	+	–	–	–	–	–	+	–	
T. pertenue	+	–	–	–	–	–	+	–	
T. carateum	+	–	–	–	–	–	+	–	Restricted to South America
Leptospira interrogans	–	+	+	–	+	–	+	–	Over 20 serogroups
Borellia vincenti	+	–	–	–	–	–	–	–	
B. recurrentis	+	–	–	+	–	–	–	–	
B. duttoni	–	+	–	+	–	–	–	–	
B. burgdorferi	–	+	–	+	–	–	–	–	

303 Spirochaetes. Sources and transmission of bacteria.

SPIROCHAETES
IDENTIFYING CHARACTERISTICS

Organism	Microscopy	Other tests for identification
Treponema pallidum T. pertenue T. carateum	Coiled, straight spirochaetes seen in dark field of specimen from ulcers	Diagnosis usually by cardiolipin and trepanomal antibody tests
Leptospira interrogans	Tightly coiled with hooked ends seen by dark-field microscopy of urine or CSF	Diagnosis usually by serological tests
Borellia vincenti	Gram –ve wavy shape in smears	
B. recurrentis B. duttoni	Wavy-shaped spirochaetes seen in Giemsa blood stains	Diagnosis usually from blood film and clinical symptoms
B. burgdorferi		Diagnosis usually by serological tests

304 Spirochaetes. Identifying characteristics.

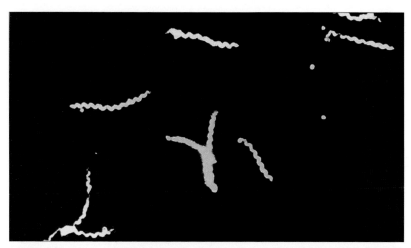

305 Dark-field microscopy of *Treponema pallidum*. *Treponema pallidum* appears as straight, tightly coiled spirochaetes on dark-field microscopy. *(Dark-field microscopy, ×1000)*

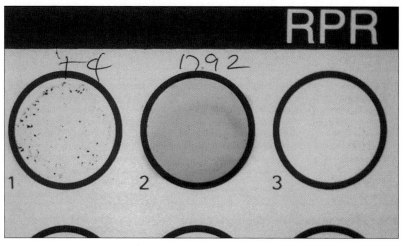

306 Rapid plasma reagin (RPR) test for syphilis. The RPR is a cardiolipin (non-treponemal) antibody test for syphilis, positive in the early stages of the disease. The patient's serum is mixed with commercially prepared carbon-linked cardiolipin antigen. A positive serum shows clumping of the antigen particles. *(Clumping of particles observed after 4 min)*

Leptospira interrogans, the cause of leptospirosis, can be demonstrated by dark-field microscopy, silver staining and immunofluorescence (**307**). *Borellia recurrentis*, the cause of relapsing fever, can be seen in Giemsa stains of blood films from infected patients (**308**). Serological tests are used in the

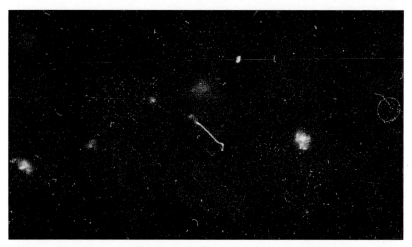

307 Dark-field microscopy of *Leptospira interrogans*. Leptospira are tightly coiled spirochaetes, characteristically with hooked ends. A zoonosis, they cause leptospirosis or Weil's disease in humans. *(Dark-field microscopy, ×1000)*

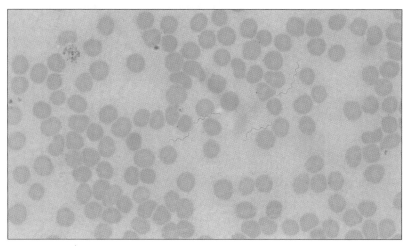

308 Giemsa stain of *Borrelia recurrentis* from the blood of a patient with relapsing fever. *Borrelia* are relatively large, wavy spirochaetes, appearing mauve-red on Giemsa staining. *(Giemsa stain, ×1000)*

RICKETTSIA AND COXIELLA INFECTIONS

Organism	Major infection	Less common infection	Vaccine preventable?	Incubation period	Period of infectivity
Rickettsia typhi	Flea-borne (murine) typhus	–	–	1–2 weeks	Not from infected cases
R. prowazekii	Louse-borne typhus	–	(+)	1–2 weeks	Infective for lice in febrile period
R. tsutsugamaushi	Scrub (mite-borne) typhus	–	–	6–21 days	Not person-to-person
R. rickettsii	Rocky-mountain spotted fever	–	–	3–14 days	Ticks up to 18 months
Coxiella burnetii	'Q fever', pneumonitis	Endocarditis	+/–	2–3 weeks	–

309a   Rickettsia and Coxiella. Infections.

RICKETTSIA AND COXIELLA SOURCES AND TRANSMISSION OF BACTERIA

Organism	Reservoir			Transmission					Comments
	Man	Animal	Env.	Insect	Feco-oral	Droplet	Direct	Nosocomial	
Rickettsia typhi	–	+	–	+ (flea)	–	–	+	–	
R. prowazeki	+	–	–	+ (louse)	–	–	–	–	
R. tsutsugamushi	+	+	–	+ (mite)	–	–	–	–	
R. rickettsii	–	+	–	+ (tick)	–	–	–	–	
Coxiella burnetii	–	+	–	–	+/–	+	–	–	

309b   Rickettsia and Coxiella. Sources and transmission of bacteria.

RICKETTSIA AND COXIELLA IDENTIFYING CHARACTERISTICS

Organism	Microscopy	Serology	Well-Felix reaction		
			OX-19	OX-2	OX-K
Rickettsia typhi	Pleomorphic	Diagnosis serological by complement fixation test or Weil-Felix reaction	+	+/–	–
R. prowazekii			+	+/–	–
R. tsutsugamushi			–	–	+/–
R. ricketsii			+	+	–
Coxiella burnetii			–	–	–

309c   Rickettsia and Coxiella. Identifying characteristics.

diagnosis of rickettsial infections. The Weil–Felix test is a non-specific test based on the agglutination of certain *Proteus vulgaris* strains by antibodies to rickettsia (**310**). Q fever, caused by *Coxiella burnetii*, may be diagnosed by microtitre complement fixation tests (**311**).

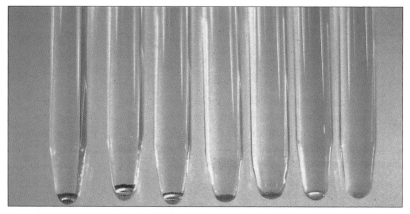

310 The Weil–Felix reaction in rickettsial infections. Antibodies to rickettsiae cross-react with certain strains of *Proteus vulgaris* and *P. mirabilis*. The patient's serum is incubated with commercially prepared, stained antigen suspensions and agglutination observed. Serial dilutions of serum are made from 1:20 to 1:280. The patient's serum shows a positive reaction (in this case to *P. vulgaris* OX-19 antigen) at a titre of 1:320. *(4 h incubation at 50ºC)*

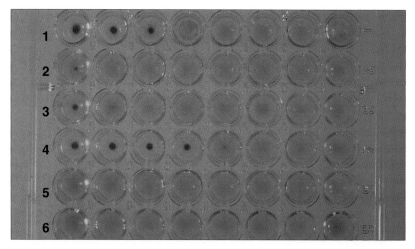

311 Microtitre complement fixation test in the diagnosis of a *Coxiella burnetii* infection. Row 4 is a serial dilution of the patient's serum against the phase I antigen of *Coxiella burnetii* showing a positive result up to a titre of 1:64 (dilutions 1:8–1:512, control). *(18 h incubation at 4ºC, red cells added and incubated for 30 min at 37ºC)*

■ CHLAMYDIACEAE

The Chlamydiaceae, summarized in **312** and **313**, are obligate intracellular bacteria. They have both DNA and RNA, and a cell wall, and divide by binary fission. They enter their host cell by endocytosis and replicate within the endosome to form a large inclusion (**314**). They exist in two forms, the

CHLAMYDIA INFECTIONS					
Organism	**Major infection**	**Less common infection**	**Vaccine preventable?**	**Incubation period**	**Period of infectivity**
Chlamydia psittaci	Psittacosis	Infections in pregnancy (ovine strains)	–	4–15 days	Person-to-person rare
C. trachomatis A–C	Trachoma	–	–	5–12 days	Years if not treated
C. trachomatis D–K	Sexually transmitted disease, urethritis, pelvic inflammatory disease, neonatal pneumonia/ophthalmia	–	–	7–14 days	?
C. trachomatis L1–L3	Lympho-granuloma venereum	–	–	3–30 days	? Years
C. pneumoniae (TWAR)	Atypical pneumonia	Otitis media	–	>10 days	? Months

312a *Chlamydia.* Infections.

CHLAMYDIA SOURCES AND TRANSMISSION OF BACTERIA									
	Reservoir			**Transmission**					
Organism	**Man**	**Animal**	**Env.**	**Insect**	**Feco-oral**	**Droplet**	**Direct**	**Nosocomial**	**Comments**
Chlamydia psittaci	–	+	–	–	+	+	–	–	
C. trachomatis A–C	+	–	–	+	–	+	+	–	
C. trachomatis D–K	+	–	–	–	–	–	+	–	
C. trachomatis L	+	–	–	–	–	–	+	–	
C. pneumoniae	+	–	–	–	–	+	+	–	

312b *Chlamydia.* Sources and transmission of bacteria.

CHLAMYDIA IDENTIFYING CHARACTERISTICS			
Organism	Culture	Antigen/genome detection	Serology
Chlamydia psittaci C. trachomatis C. pneumoniae	Fertile hen's eggs McCoy cells McCoy cells, but culture difficult	IFAT/ELISA IFAT/ELISA/PCR IFAT/PCR	Complement fixation test Micro-immune fluorescence Micro-immune fluorescence
IFAT = immunofluorescent antigen test. ELISA = enzyme-linked immunosorbent assay. PCR = polymerase chain reaction.			

313 *Chlamydia.* Identifying characteristics.

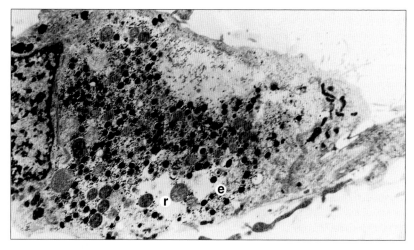

314 *Chlamydia trachomatis* showing inclusion bodies. Thin-section electron micrograph of a McCoy cell containing a large *C. trachomatis* inclusion. The small, electron-dense forms are elementary bodies **(e)** and the larger forms are reticulate **(r)** bodies.

elementary body, which is small and electron dense, and is the extracellular infective form, and the larger more fragile reticulate body, which is the replicating form found only in inclusions.

There are three main species pathogenic for man.

Chlamydia psittaci

Despite its name, this bacterium infects a large variety of species as well as psittacine birds (parrots, budgerigars). *Chlamydia psittaci* is a cause of primary atypical pneumonia usually acquired from birds. Another serovar of *C. psittaci*, the ewe abortion agent, is a rare cause of early abortion, stillbirth and fetal septicemia. Diagnosis is by demonstration of the agent in tissue by immunofluorescence or serology. Culture is by inoculation into the yolk sac of fertile hen's eggs and requires special containment facilities.

Chlamydia trachomatis

Chlamydia trachomatis strains A–C cause trachoma, which is the most common infective cause of blindness in developing countries. *Chlamydia trachomatis* strains D–K cause a sexually transmitted infection throughout the world. Infection can be silent (especially in women) but can cause urethritis, cervicitis, epididymitis (in males) and ascend to cause pelvic inflammatory disease in women. It is now the most common sexually transmitted infection since gonorrhea has receded. If a neonate is born through an infected cervix, it has a 50% chance of developing ophthalmia neonatorum, which may subsequently lead to pneumonia.

Diagnosis can be by culture in epithelial cells (e.g. McCoy), but this takes up to 72 h for the characteristic inclusions to be visible (**315**). More rapid diagnosis is by ELISA and immunofluorescent antigen test (**316**). The gold standard for diagnosis is now, however, the automated polymerase chain reaction (**85**).

Chlamydia pneumoniae

This recently discovered pathogen was originally called the TWAR (*T*ai*w*an, *a*cute *r*espiratory) agent. It is a cause of primary atypical pneumonia, especially in adolescents and young adults. It has recently been associated

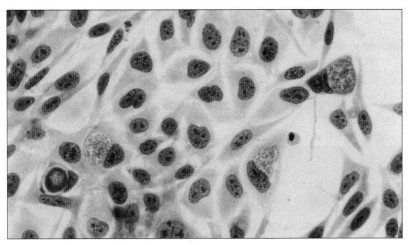

315 *Chlamydia trachomatis* **cultured on McCoy cells.** Giemsa-stained McCoy cells containing large chlamydial inclusions partially obscuring the nuclei. *(Giemsa stain, ×1000)*

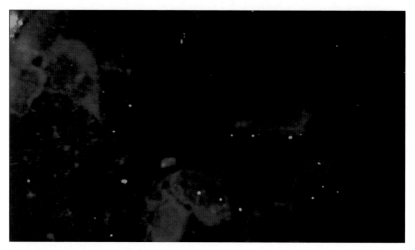

316 *Chlamydia trachomatis,* **immunofluorescence.** Indirect immunofluorescence of a cervical smear showing apple-green fluorescent *C. trachomatis* elementary bodies. *(Fluorescence microscopy, ×1000)*

with the development of coronary heart disease. Diagnosis is by serology, culture or genome detection by polymerase chain reaction.

■ ANTIMICROBIAL AGENTS AND ANTIMICROBIAL RESISTANCE
Abbreviations used for antibiotics

AMC	Augmentin
AML	Amoxycillin
C	Chloramphenicol
CAZ	Ceftazidime
CE	Cefaclor
CIP	Ciprofloxacin
CN	Gentamicin
CTX	Cefotaxime
F	Nitrofurantoin
MET	Methicillin
MTZ	Metronidazole
NA	Nalidixic acid
OX	Oxacillin
P	Penicillin
RD	Rifampicin
RL	Sulfamethoxazole
T	Tetracycline
VA	Vancomycin
W	Trimethoprim

Strictly speaking, an antibiotic is an antimicrobial compound derived from a living organism, whereas the term 'antimicrobial' encompasses both antibiotics and synthetic and semi-synthetic molecules (**317**). In practice, the terms are often used interchangeably. The mechanisms by which important groups of antimicrobials inhibit bacterial growth is shown in **318**.

By extracting, purifying and administering antimicrobials in large quantities to a large number of patients, we have greatly speeded up bacterial evolution over the past 60 or so years. The evolutionary pressure of antimicrobial agents has driven the selection of bacteria resistant to the drugs. This has occurred to such an extent that some have heralded this as the end of the antibiotic era.

Some bacteria may be intrinsically resistant to particular antibiotics, or they may acquire resistance through genetic transfer. Examples of bacterial resistance mechanisms are shown in **319**.

Trimethoprim inhibits the bacterial enzyme dihydrofolate reductase (DHFR). This enzyme is the final part of the pathway to synthesize folic acid, which bacteria cannot acquire exogenously. Folic acid is needed by the bacteria to synthesize new nucleotides so, by inhibiting DHFR, bacteria cannot make new DNA or RNA and thus die. Resistance is imparted by the production of a mutated DHFR with far lower affinity for trimethoprim. This mechanism of resistance is particularly important among enterobacteria.

THE ANTIBIOTIC ERA			
1928	Fleming	*Penicillium notatum*	Penicillins
1935	Domagk	Synthetic	Sulfonamides
1941	Forey and Chain	*Penicillium notatum*	Penicillin G
1944	Duggan	*Streptomyces aureofaciens*	Tetracyclines
1945	Waksman	*Streptomyces griseus*	Streptomycin
1945	Brotzu	*Cephalosporium* spp	Cephalosporins
1947	Ehrlich	*Streptomyces venezuelae*	Chloramphenicol
1952	McGuire	*Streptomyces erythreus*	Erythromycin
1956	McCormick	*Streptomyces orientalis*	Vancomycin
1957	Rolinson	Semi-synthetic	6-Amino penicilloic acid
1959	Cosar	Synthetic	Metronidazole
1962	Lescher	Synthetic	Nalidixic acid
1962	Roth	Synthetic	Trimethoprim
1964	Weinstein	*Micromonospora* spp	Gentamicin
1966	Bergamini	*Streptomyces mediterranei*	Rifampicin
1978	Sykes	*Chromobacterium violaceum*	Monobactams
1978	Various	*Streptomyces pristinaespiralis*	Streptogramins
1983	Various	*Streptomyces roseosporus*	Daptomycin
1984	Various	Synthetic	Fluoroquinolones
1987	Slee	Synthetic	Oxazolidinone
1999	Various	Semi-synthetic	Ketolides

317 The antibiotic era.

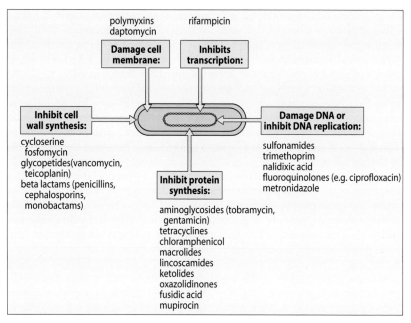

318 Mechanisms of antimicrobial action against bacteria.

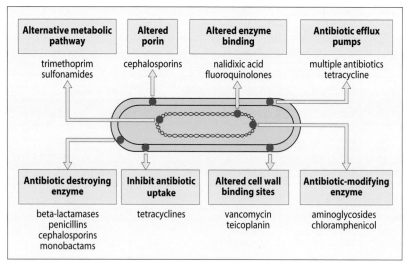

319 Mechanisms of bacterial resistance to antimicrobials.

The fluoroquinolones inhibit the packaging of DNA during replication. DNA gyrase enzymes cut and rejoin DNA strands after supercoiling it. The fluoroquinolones bind to these enzymes, inhibiting their activity. Resistance occurs when mutations in genes encoding the enzymes prevent binding and inhibition. In Gram-negative bacteria, hydrophilic antimicrobials must traverse the bacterial outer membrane to gain access to their target. They most often gain access through pores in the outer membranes made up of proteins called porins. Mutants have been described in which alterations in porins alter the size and structure of the porin so that large, bulky molecules such as cephalosporins can no longer gain entry. Finally, a recently discovered multiple antibiotic resistance mechanism imparts resistance to many antimicrobials at once by pumping them out of the bacterium. Such efflux pumps have also been shown to render bacteria resistance to tetracyclines.

Within the laboratory, antimicrobial sensitivity testing is most commonly carried out by a disc diffusion method. In Stoke's method, plates are usually inoculated so that the test isolate and a known, fully sensitive control organism can be compared. After inoculation of the plates, antimicrobial-containing discs are placed at the interface of the test and control inocula. The plates are incubated overnight and the growth inhibition zones compared between the test and control strains. In most cases, a resistant strain is defined as growing adjacent to a disc or having a zone radius less than 2 mm. **320** shows the association between zone size and antibiotic concentration. Examples of disc sensitivity testing are shown for *S. aureus* (**321**) and *E. coli* (**322**). More standardized methods, such as those of the NCCLS or BSAC, have now been introduced whereby standardized media, bacterial inocula and incubation conditions are used. The zone of inhibition size is measured and then related to the minimum inhibitory concentration (MIC) of the particular antimicrobial agent (**323**).

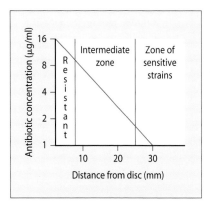

320 Regression line showing the association between distance from the antibiotic disc, antibiotic concentration and zone size for bacteria with different minimum inhibitory concentrations (MIC). The regression line represents the decreasing antibiotic concentration with distance from the disc. Zone size depends on the MIC and is usually compared with that of a known sensitive strain.

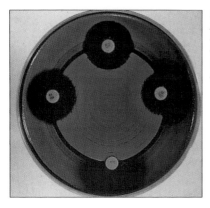

321 Disc sensitivity testing for
Staphylococcus aureus. The outer rim is a
control *S. aureus* NCTC 6571 sensitive to P, F,
CE and CN. Centrally, *S. aureus* is resistant to P.
It is sensitive to the other antimicrobials. *(DST
agar with 5% lysed blood, 18 h at 37ºC)*

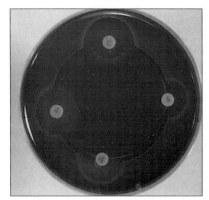

322 Sensitive and resistant *Escherichia coli*
strains. The outer rim is a control *E. coli* NCTC
sensitive to AML, W, F, and NA showing
inhibition zones around each antimicrobial
disc. An *E. coli* from a clinical specimen is
plated centrally showing sensitivity to F and
NA and resistance (no inhibition zones) to AML
and W. *(DST agar with 5% lysed blood, 18 h at
37ºC)*

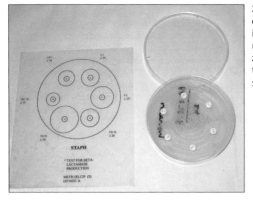

**323 An example of BSAC disc
diffusion testing.** The zone of
inhibition is directly related to the
minimum inhibitory concentration
zone of the antimicrobial. The
template is used to measure zone
sizes.

Resistance to penicillins and related antibiotics is often due to the production by the bacteria of beta lactamase enzymes that destroy the beta lactam ring. **324** shows an *E. coli* resistant to amoxycillin as a result of beta lactamase production, with no inhibition zone around the amoxycillin disc. The antimicrobial agent augmentin contains amoxycillin and the beta lactamase inhibitor clavulanic acid. The beta lactamase is thus inhibited, and the *E. coli* is rendered sensitive to the amoxycillin in the disc, resulting in a zone of inhibition. If a beta lactamase-producing organism fails to produce sufficient enzyme to destroy the concentration of antibiotic near the disc, an inhibition zone will occur, but the colonies at the edge of the zone will be large, showing a 'heaped' appearance (**325**). Beta lactamase production can be demonstrated by a simple color test using the chromogenic cephalosporin nitrocefin (**326**). Methicillin resistance among strains of *S. aureus* can be determined by placing a methicillin-impregnated strip (25 µg) across streaks

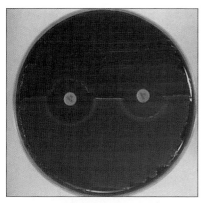

324 *Escherichia coli* showing ampicillin resistance as a result of beta lactamase production. The plate is inoculated with an *E. coli* resistant to ampicillin. The strain is sensitive to augmentin. Augmentin is an agent containing ampicillin and the beta lactamase inhibitor clavulanic acid. *(DST agar with 5% lysed blood, 18 h at 37ºC)*

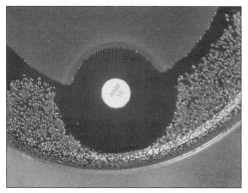

325 *Escherichia coli* demonstrating amoxycillin resistance as a result of beta lactamase production. The outer rim is a fully sensitive *E. coli*. The resistant strain does show an inhibition zone, but it is smaller and the edge has a 'heaped' appearance. *(DST agar with 5% lysed blood, 18 h at 37ºC)*

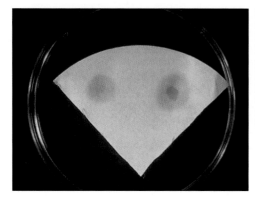

326 Chromogenic cephalosporin (nitrocefin) test to demonstrate beta lactamase production. Nitrocefin changes color from yellow to red in the presence of beta lactamase. A beta lactamase-producing, ampicillin-resistant strain of *Haemophilus influenzae* has been scraped on to the strip, which shows the red color after 60 seconds.

of the test isolate and known methicillin-sensitive and resistant strains for comparison (**327**).

Penicillin resistance is an increasing clinical problem in *S. pneumoniae* and is caused by alterations in penicillin-binding proteins. It has been shown that a 1 μg oxacillin disc gives the most reproducible in vivo result (**328**). Disc sensitivity testing for *H. influenzae*, *N. meningitidis* and *N. gonorrhoeae* are shown in **329–331**.

Clinical isolates of *Ps. aeruginosa* are frequently resistant to multiple antimicrobial agents. **332** shows *Ps. aeruginosa* resistant to gentamicin and cefotaxime. There have been recent reports of *Enterococcus faecium* with a low or even high level resistance to vancomycin (**333**).

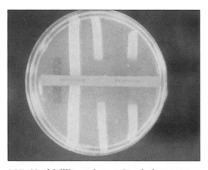

327 Methicillin-resistant *Staphylococcus aureus*. The strip contains 25 μg methicillin. For sensitive strains, there is a zone of no growth on either side of the strip. The methicillin-resistant *S. aureus* grows up to the strip. *(Columbia agar, 18 h at 37ºC)*

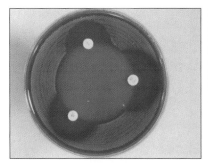

328 Penicillin-resistant *Streptococcus pneumoniae*. The outer rim is inoculated with a sensitive control *S. aureus*. Penicillin-resistant strains of *S. pneumoniae* are demonstrated using a 1 μg oxacillin disc. The resistant *S. pneumoniae* plated centrally is penicillin and erythromycin resistant. *(Chocolate agar, 18 h at 37ºC)*

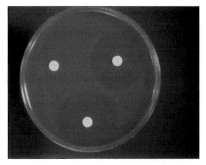

329 *Haemophilus influenzae*, ampicillin resistance. Disc sensitivity plate showing *H. influenzae* resistant to ampicillin but sensitive to chloramphenicol and cefotaxime. *(Chocolate agar, 18 h at 37ºC)*

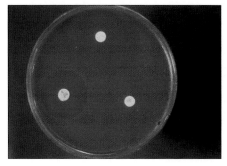

330 *Neisseria meningitidis* sensitivity. Disc sensitivity showing *N. meningitidis* sensitive to penicillin and rifampicin but resistant to sulfonamide. *(Chocolate agar, 18 h at 37ºC)*

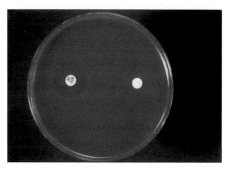

331 *Neisseria gonorrhoeae* **resistant to penicillin.** Disc sensitivity showing *N. gonorrhoeae* resistant to penicillin and sensitive to spectinomycin. *(Chocolate agar, 18 h at 37°C)*

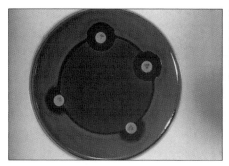

332 *Pseudomonas aeruginosa* **sensitivity testing.** The outer rim is a *Ps. aeruginosa* control (NCTC 10662) sensitive to CTX, CN, CIP, CAZ. The test sample shows resistance to cefotaxime and gentamicin. *(DST agar with 5% lysed blood, 18 h at 37°C)*

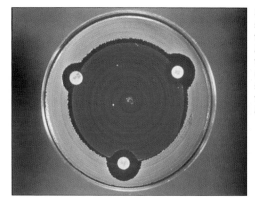

333 *Enterococcus faecalis* **showing resistance to vancomycin.** Some strains of *E. faecalis* show low-level resistance to vancomycin. The strain is resistant to the 5 µg disc but sensitive to the 30 µg disc and to teicoplanin. *(DST agar with 5% lysed blood, 18 h at 37°C)*

When a large number of isolates is to be tested for antimicrobial sensitivity, the use of agar plates incorporating antibiotics of known concentrations is useful. The antibiotic concentration is chosen as a 'break point' below which sensitive strains will grow but above which only resistant strains will grow (**334**).

Disc sensitivity testing gives only a qualitative guide to the sensitivity or resistance of an isolate. More quantitative methods enable the determination of the MIC and minimum bactericidal concentration (MBC) of an antimicrobial against a clinical isolate. These determinations are important in serious infections such as endocarditis and when using antimicrobials with a dose-related toxicity. **335** shows the tube method for determining MIC, and **336** MBC determination.

In clinical practice, a knowledge of synergy and antagonism between antimicrobial agents is important. **337** demonstrates synergy between trimethoprim and a sulfonamide, two agents that work at different sites of bacterial nucleic acid synthesis. Antagonism between nalidixic acid and nitrofurantoin is shown in **338**. Antagonism between antimicrobials may arise through the induction of class I beta lactamase by one beta lactam reducing the effect of a second beta lactam (**339**). Synergistic activity is important in clinical practice, a combination of antimicrobials possibly allowing a lower dose of a potentially toxic agent to be used. **340** demonstrates the synergistic effects of gentamicin and penicillin.

In severe infections, it is useful to determine the serum bactericidal activity against the patient's clinical isolate. Serum samples are taken pre-dose and generally 1 h post-dose, and the maximum serum dilution giving inhibitory and bactericidal activity is determined (**341, 342**). A minimum bactericidal dilution of 1:8 in the peak serum sample is regarded as adequate, although some studies suggest that a dilution in excess of 1:32 may be necessary for cure.

An additional investigation to determine the probable in vivo activity of an antimicrobial agent, and to monitor toxic levels, is to assay the antimicrobial

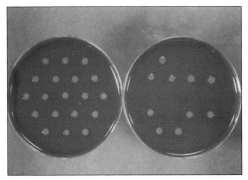

334 Break-point sensitivity testing of *Escherichia coli* to amoxycillin. Test strains are inoculated on to media containing different concentrations of amoxycillin using a multipoint inoculator. After overnight incubation, the presence or absence of growth is noted. (*DST agar with 5% lysed blood. Plate amoxycillin concentrations: left, 1 μg/ml; right, 8 μg/ml*)

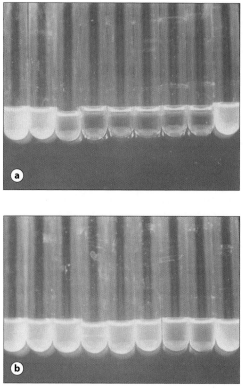

335 Tube minimum inhibitory concentration (MIC) of two *Escherichia coli* isolates to ampicillin. Serial dilutions of ampicillin from 0.5 µg/ml to 64 µg/ml are prepared. 1 ml of the test organism suspension is added to each tube. After overnight incubation, visual turbidity is noted. The MIC is the lowest antibiotic concentration in which there is no visible growth. In the upper row **(a)**, the MIC is 2 µg/ml. In the lower row **(b)**, the MIC is 32 µg/ml. *(Ampicillin concentrations (µg/ml) left to right: 0.5, 1, 2, 4, 8, 16, 32, 64, 0 (control))*

concentration in the serum. **343** shows microbiological plate assays to determine the pre- and post-dose levels of gentamicin.

Acquired resistance to antimicrobials is an increasing problem, leading some to prophesy the end of the antibiotic era. Resistance may be acquired by chromosomal mutation, as is the case for acquired resistance to fluoroquinolones. In general, these resistances do not transfer to other bacteria; i.e they are clonal. Resistance to most, if not all, antimicrobials can, however, be transferred across species and genera, and within bacterial species. This occurs if the antimicrobial resistance genes are encoded on mobile genetic elements such as plasmids, transposons or integrons. Plasmids are supercoiled extrachromosomal loops of DNA. Transposons and integrons are sets of genes that can be excised from DNA (chromosome or plasmid) and re-inserted into bacterial plasmids or chromosomes, either site-specifically (integrons) or at random (transposons). The sequential addition of

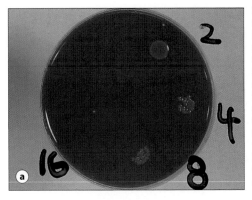

336 Minimum bactericidal concentration (MBC) of *Escherichia coli* **to ampicillin.** From each of the non-turbid tubes of the minimum inhibitory concentration (MIC) test, 20 µl is spotted on to a section of blood agar plate and incubated overnight. The lowest concentration giving no growth on the plate is the MBC. For the isolate with the MIC of 2 µg/ml, the MBC is 16 µg/ml **(a)**. For the isolate with the MIC of 32 µg/ml, the MBC is greater than 64 µg/ml **(b)**. *(Blood agar, 18 h at 37ºC)*

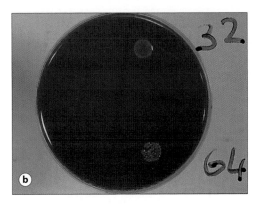

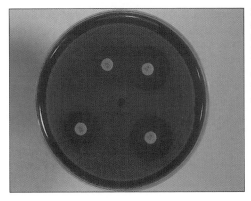

337 Demonstration of antimicrobial synergy. The test shows synergy of action by trimethoprim and sulfamethoxazole. The zone size is increased in the area between the discs where both antibiotics are present. *(Escherichia coli on DST agar with 5% lysed blood, 18 h at 37ºC)*

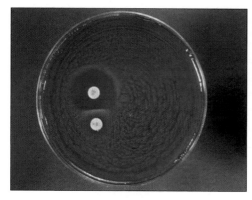

338 Demonstration of antimicrobial antagonism. The test shows antagonism of antimicrobial action by nalidixic acid and nitrofurantoin. The zone size is decreased in the area between the discs where both antibiotics are present. *(Proteus vulgaris on CLED agar, 18 h at 37°C)*

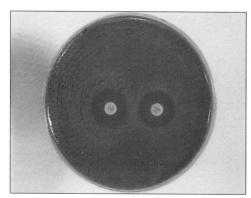

339 Induction of beta lactamase production. Imipenem induces beta lactamase production in *Pseudomonas aeruginosa*, reducing the zone size to piperacillin. *(DST agar with 5% lysed blood, 18 h at 37°C)*

transposons and or integrons (jumping genes) is responsible for the assembly of large multiresistance plasmids. DNA, usually in the form of plasmids, can move from bacterium to bacterium by conjugation (**344**) in a process analogous to mating, which is important in Gram-negative bacteria. Transduction (**345**) is the process by which resistance genes are transferred between bacteria by bacterial viruses (bacteriophages, **346**). This is particularly important for the movement of beta lactamase genes between *S. aureus* strains. Transduction involves the movement of DNA directly between bacteria and is important only for transformation-competent bacteria such as streptococci and *Neisseria* spp.

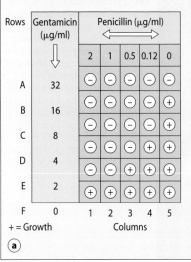

Rows	Gentamicin (μg/ml) ⬇	Penicillin (μg/ml) ⬅⟶				
		2	1	0.5	0.12	0
A	32	−	−	−	−	−
B	16	−	−	−	−	+
C	8	−	−	−	−	+
D	4	−	−	−	+	+
E	2	−	−	+	+	+
F	0	+	+	+	+	+
		1	2	3	4	5

+ = Growth   Columns

(a)

340 Antimicrobial agents in combination.
Each well in the plate contains a different combination of penicillin and gentamicin, shown in **a**. Row F shows growth at all concentrations of penicillin in the absence of gentamicin. Column 5 shows growth at all concentrations of gentamicin, except at 32 μg/ml, in the absence of penicillin. The two antimicrobials work synergistically, growth being inhibited at a gentamicin concentration of 2 μg/ml in the presence of 1 μg/ml of penicillin **(b)**.

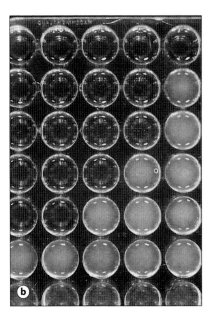

(b)

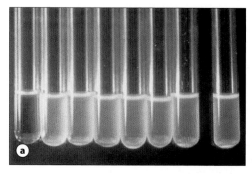

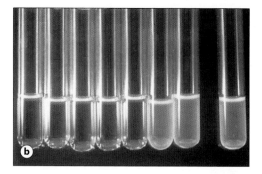

341 Back titration to determine antimicrobial activity in serum. Pre- and post-dose blood samples are taken from the patient during antimicrobial therapy. The serum is serially diluted and inoculated with 1 ml of a broth culture of the patient's isolate, and the tubes are incubated overnight. **a** and **b** show that the pre-dose minimum inhibitory dilution is 1:2, and the post-dose equivalent 1:32. *(Broth dilutions, left to right – 1:2, 1:4, 1:8, 1:16, 1:32, 1:64, 1:128, control)*

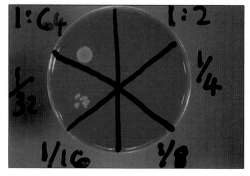

342 Minimum bactericidal dilution (MBD). For the post-dose situation, 20 μl samples from tubes with no growth have been spotted on to blood agar and incubated overnight to determine the MBD, which is 1:16. *(Blood agar, 18 h at 37°C)*

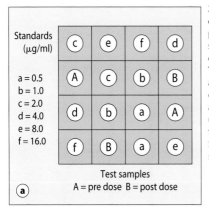

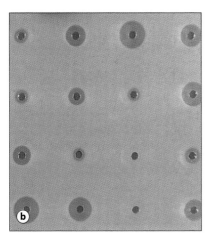

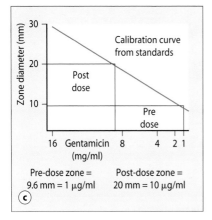

343 Plate assay to determine the blood concentration of gentamicin. The plate is poured with isosenitest agar, which is, after setting, inoculated with a 1:50 dilution of an overnight broth culture of *Klebsiella edwardsii*. The wells are cut and gentamicin standards and the test sample added as in **a**. After overnight incubation (**b**), the inhibition zones are measured and a standard curve drawn (**c**). The concentration of gentamicin in the test samples is determined from the graph. Sample A concentration is 1 µg/ml and that of sample B 10 µg/ml.

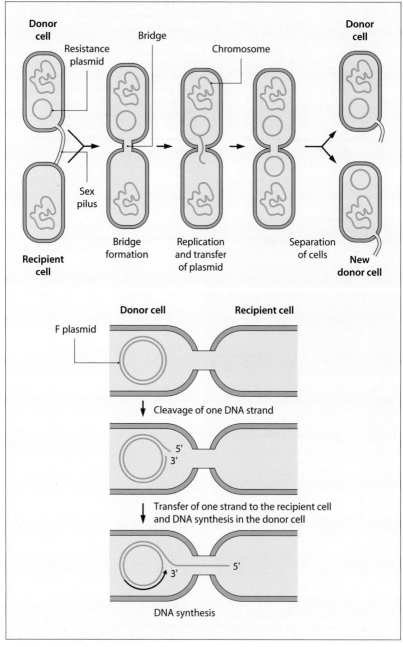

344   Bacterial conjugation transferring a resistance plasmid.

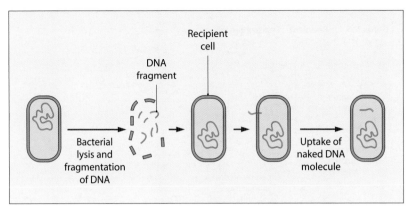

345 Transduction.

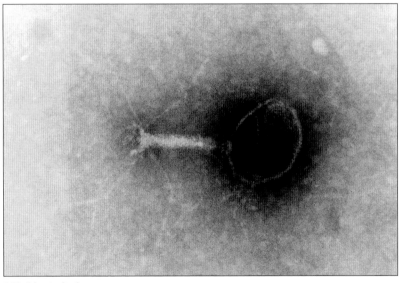

346 A bacteriophage.

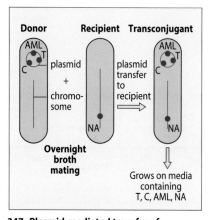

347 Plasmid-mediated transfer of antimicrobial resistance genes. The donor is resistant to ampicillin, tetracycline and chloramphenicol, and sensitive to nalidixic acid. The recipient *Escherichia coli* K12 is resistant only to nalidixic acid. The transconjugant is resistant to all four antimicrobial agents.

The remaining figures in this section describe the transfer of antimicrobial resistance determinants. **347** describes the principle of the plasmid-mediated transfer of resistance genes. In the laboratory, exponential cultures of a multiply resistant donor and a suitable recipient, containing a chromosomally located resistance marker, are incubated overnight and plated on to a medium containing the recipient marker antibiotic and one of the antibiotics to which the donor is resistant. Transconjugants (the recipient strain now containing plasmid-borne genes from the donor) will grow on the selective plate. **348** demonstrates resistance transfer in *E. coli*. **349** is a gel showing the plasmid profiles of donors and recipients, demonstrating the transferred plasmids.

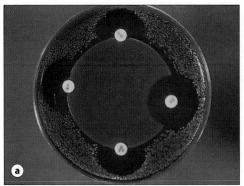

348 Transfer of resistance by bacterial conjugation. The donor *Escherichia coli* isolate **(a)** is sensitive to NA and resistant to AML, T and C. The recipient is a laboratory strain (*E. coli*, K12, NA^R) sensitive to AML, T and C with chromosomally located NA resistance **(b)**. **c** The transconjugant, which is resistant to all four antibiotics.

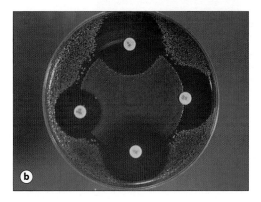

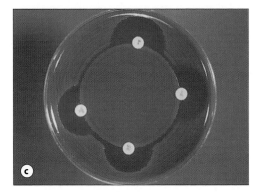

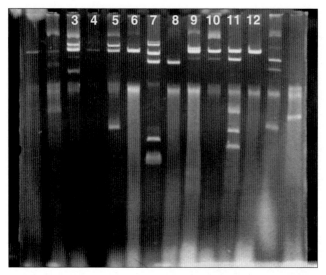

349 Agarose gel electrophoresis showing the transfer of antimicrobial resistant plasmids. Lanes 3–12 show alternate donors and transconjugants demonstrating plasmid transfer. As an example, lane 3 is a donor with four plasmids (above the broad band of chromosomal DNA). Lane 4 is the transconjugant, which has one plasmid from the donor. *(DNA extraction by SDS lysis and ethanol precipitation. 0.7% agarose gel electrophoresis. Stained with ethidium bromide.)*

Chapter 5

DIAGNOSTIC, EPIDEMIOLOGICAL AND MOLECULAR TECHNOLOGIES

Diagnostic bacteriology traditionally involved the culture of a clinical sample on media designed to support the growth of pathogens likely to cause infection at the particular anatomical site. This is, of necessity, time-consuming in that it depends upon the time taken for bacteria to grow and thus become detectable. There are now ways to speed up detection. Blood is normally sterile, and detecting bacteria in the blood (bacteremia) means there is a serious infection. Blood is taken under sterile conditions, 5–10 ml (from adults) being placed into an enriched broth containing an anti-coagulant. This would once have been incubated at 37°C for up to 2 weeks and examined daily for evidence of bacterial growth. Now, however, the process has been automated such that positive blood cultures can be detected within 12 h of incubation. These systems depend upon the detection of bacterial metabolism, for example carbon dioxide or nitrogen production (**350**).

Although a large number of molecular biological techniques are used in diagnostic virology, they are in their infancy in diagnostic bacteriology. Part of the problem is that catch-all techniques such as the amplification and sequencing of 16S rRNA genes, which will allow the precise identification of bacteria, are of value only for the diagnosis of infection in normally sterile sites. Otherwise the normal flora of, for example, the intestinal tract would drown out any signals from the pathogens. A pathogen-specific polymerase chain reaction (PCR) is used, for example, to detect *Chlamydia*, gonococci, meningococci or epidemic *Pseudomonas aeruginosa* in sputum from patients with cystic fibrosis (**351**). However, only a limited number of pathogens can be detected at once even with multiplex PCR. This problem is being addressed by use of microarray technology (**352**). In this, probes for up to 200 000 different genes (from different pathogens) are printed on to glass slides and the presence of a pathogen's specific DNA is detected by hybridization.

In certain infections, bacteria form biofilms that can make both laboratory diagnosis and therapy difficult. Such biofilms occur naturally in the oral cavity with consortia of bacteria sticking to each other, teeth and the mucosa. Biofilms are of particular importance in implant infections and in the lung in

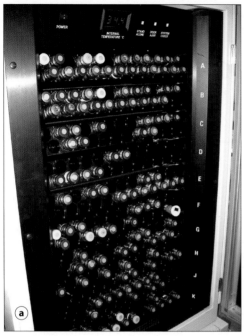

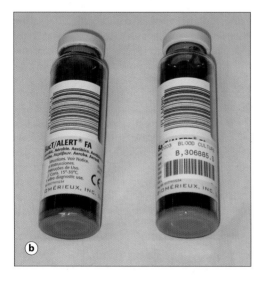

350 An automated blood culture machine (a) and blood culture bottles (b). The bottle on the right gives a positive signal (yellow base).

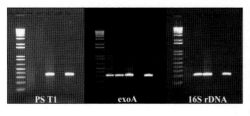

351 A polymerase chain reaction (PCR) for the detection of an epidemic strain of *Ps. aeruginosa* in a cystic fibrosis patient. Primers for 16s RNA (to detect the presence of bacteria), exotoxin A (to detect *Ps. aeruginosa*) and a gene specific to an epidemic strain of *Ps. aerugonisa* are used and, after PCR, electrophoresed on an agarose gel to separate the products.

352 A microarray. The binding of pathogen DNA to the microarray is indicated by intensity of color.

cystic fibrosis. Plastic implantable material such as central venous catheters, heart valves and ventriculo-peritoneal shunts are prone to colonization/ infection with coagulase-negative staphylococci, principally *Staphylococcus epidermidis*. The bacteria usually gain access to the implant at the time of insertion in the case of ventriculo-peritoneal shunts and are derived from either the patient's or the operating theatre staff's skin flora. The bacteria stick to the plastic by electrostatic, hydrophobic or van der Waals forces. They then grow and release extracellular slime until a large number are embedded as a biofilm in the slime (**353**). In the biofilm, they grow slowly and are protected from both body defenses and antimicrobial agents. Diagnosis can be difficult unless bacteria become detached (planktonic) from the biofilm. The cystic fibrosis bronchial tree is particularly prone to infection with *Ps. aeruginosa* and *Burkholderia cenocepacia*. In such circum-stances, they exist as biofilms attached to the respiratory mucosa. The process by which this occurs is called quorum sensing (**354**). In this, the bacteria, once they have reached a sufficiently high density, send out small molecular-weight signaling molecules (homoserine lactones). These tell the

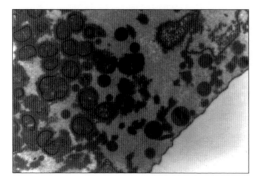

353 Thin-section electron micrograph of a ventriculo-peritoneal shunt with a biofilm of *Staphylococcus epidermidis*.

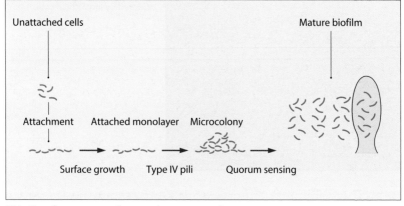

354 *Pseudomonas aeruginosa* **and quorum sensing.**

whole population to act in concert such that they all activate and release virulence determinants, divide in concert (usually slowly) and produce extra-cellular polysaccharides (alginate in *Ps. aeruginosa*). They thus act like a single entity in a biofilm protected from host defenses and antimicrobial agents.

In the investigation of disease outbreaks and nosocomial (hospital-associated) infections, typing the pathogen to further than species level is necessary to identify the outbreak strain. This is achieved by phenotypic or genotypic methods. Phenotypic methods include biotyping, antimicrobial resistance typing and serotyping, as discussed earlier in the text.

355 shows the bacteriophage typing of *S. aureus*. The phage type of the strain is given by the reference number of the phages that produce lysis on the plate. This can be used to type other bacteria, including *Salmonella typhi* (**356**). **357** illustrates pyocin (bacteriocin) typing of *Ps. aeruginosa*.

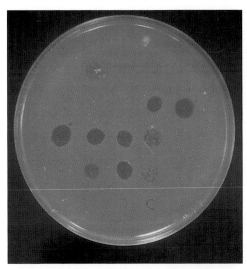

355 Bacteriophage typing of *Staphylococcus aureus*. A broth culture of *S. aureus* is seeded on to the plate, and specific phages are spotted on a grid system. After overnight incubation, lysis indicates the phage type of the *S. aureus* stain. *(Nutrient agar, 18 h at 37°C)*

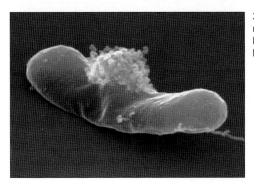

356 Scanning electron micrograph of *Salmonella typhi* being lysed by the release of bacteriophages.

Bacteriocin typing has also been used for *Shigella* spp and other Enterobacteriaceae. It is a labor-intensive method and is rarely used now that more specific and reproducible molecular techniques are available. **358** demonstrates the Dienes typing of swarming *Proteus* strains. Differing strains produce a 'ditch' of no growth between the swarming edges. Molecular and related methods are increasingly used in epidemiological studies and are becoming the gold standard. They include whole-cell and outer membrane protein typing, plasmid profiling and plasmid or chromosomal DNA restriction endonuclease typing.

359 shows whole-cell protein typing in the investigation of *Burkholderia cepacia* isolates from cases of cystic fibrosis. Additional non-DNA-based

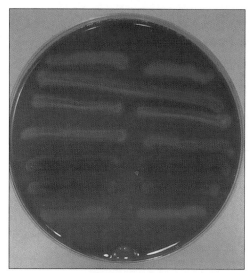

357 Pyocin typing of Pseudomonas aeruginosa. The test strain is streaked down the center of the plate. The growth is removed from the plate, which is then exposed to chloroform vapor to kill any remaining growth. Typing strains are streaked across the plate, which is again incubated. An inhibition of typing strains demonstrates the pyocin type of the test stain. (Blood agar, 18 h at 37ºC)

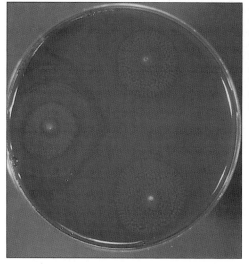

358 Dienes typing of Proteus strains. Three strains are spotted equidistantly around the periphery of the plate and incubated overnight. The two identical strains show no line of separation where the growth merges. The third, different, strain shows the line of separation. (Blood agar, 18 h at 37ºC)

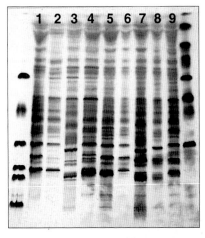

359 Whole-cell protein typing of _Burkholderia cepacia_. After cell lysis, whole cell proteins are separated by polyacrylamide gel electrophoresis and stained with Coomassie blue. The outer lanes are molecular weight standards. The protein profiles show a similarity between the strains in lanes 1–5 and lane 9.

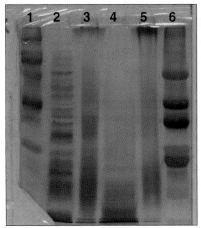

360 Demonstration of whole-cell protein (WCP), outer membrane protein (OMP) and lipopolysaccharide (LPS) typing of _Legionella_. Lanes 1 and 6 are molecular weight markers. Lane 2 shows the WCP profile. Lane 3 shows the OMP profile. Lane 4 shows LPS profiles. _(Polyacrylamide gel electrophoresis with silver stains)_

techniques include outer membrane protein analysis and lipopolysaccharide typing (**360**).

Rapid methods for small-scale DNA extraction have led to a new range of typing techniques that have a wide scope of applicability, are reproducible and provide good discrimination between strains. **361** shows plasmid profiles of _Sh. sonnei_ strains isolated from different clusters of infection and demonstrates how the profiles can distinguish among different strains.

The spread of multiply antimicrobial resistant Gram-negative bacteria is an increasing problem in hospital infection. Restriction endonuclease digests of plasmids from strains with common resistance patterns can help in defining the particular outbreak strain (**362**). Restriction endonucleases can

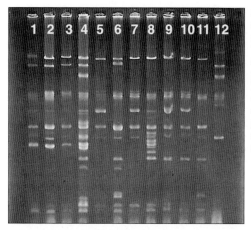

361 Plasmid profile typing of Shigella sonnei. Lane 12 shows plasmid molecular weight markers. The lanes demonstrate groups of strains with identical plasmid profiles (e.g. lanes 1–3, lanes 5 and 7, lanes 9 and 10) and others with distinct and separate profiles. *(DNA extraction by SDS lysis and ethanol precipitation. 0.7% agarose gel electrophoresis. Stained with ethidium bromide)*

362 Restriction endonuclease characterization of antimicrobial resistance plasmid from Escherichia coli. The gel shows digests of single plasmids all of molecular weight 62 MDa, using the enzyme *Pst1*. The restriction profiles of the plasmids in lanes 1, 2, 3, 4 and 7 appear identical. The plasmids in lanes 9 and 10 have a common restriction pattern but are distinguishable from the other patterns. *(DNA extraction by SDS lysis and ethanol precipitation. Enzyme digestion at 37°C for 2 h. 0.7% agarose gel electrophoresis. Stained with ethidium bromide)*

also be used to produce chromosomal DNA profiles. In this, whole-chromosomal DNA is digested with a rare cutting restriction endonuclease. Because of the large size of fragments produced, pulsed-field gel electrophoresis, with varying time/voltage parameters, is used to improve discrimination (**363**). Other technologies include multilocus sequence testing, in which the sequences of seven genes encoding enzymes not under great selection pressure (e.g. glycolytic pathway enzymes) are compared.

Disease outbreak investigations may also require environmental microbiological studies. **364** shows an example of the investigation of water quality. Fecal coliforms will grow at 44°C, and this is used to demonstrate fecal contamination.

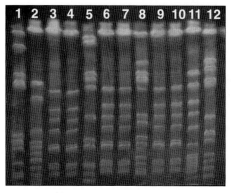

363 Pulsed-field gel electrophoresis of chromosomal DNA from different isolates of methicillin-resistant *Staphylococcus aureus* (MRSA). The gel shows chromosomal DNA from different MRSA isolates that have been digested with the restriction endonuclease *Sma*I and run by pulsed-field electrophoresis. The isolates in lanes 3, 4, 6, 7, 9 and 10 had identical profiles and were identified as an 'outbreak strain'. *(DNA extraction by cell lysis and proteinase K treatment. Electrophoresis on 1% agarose gel, angle 120º, 6 volts/cm, initial switch time 5.3 seconds, final switch time 34.9 seconds)*

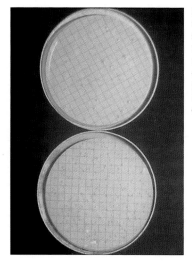

364 Membrane filtration technique for microbiological testing of water quality. Water samples of 100 ml are passed through 0.45 µm membrane filters, which are soaked in lauryl sulfate medium and incubated at 44ºC for 16 h. Fecal coliforms produce yellow colonies and the count per 100 ml is determined. Top, low coliform count. Bottom, high coliform count, suggesting considerable fecal contamination.

Chapter 6

MEDICALLY IMPORTANT FUNGI

Fungi form an extremely large kingdom, but only a small number are pathogenic for man. Fungi are eukaryotes possessing a nucleus and a cell wall composed of chitin. The major groups of pathogenic fungi are outlined in **365**. Fungi may grow in a unicellular mode (e.g. yeasts) or in a multicellular form in which cells elongate to form filaments called hyphae. The four major taxa of the true fungi (Eumycetes) are delineated by their methods of reproduction. The Zygomycetes reproduce sexually, zygotes forming by fusion of the hyphal tips. Pathogenic members of this genus include *Mucor* and *Absidia* spp. The Basidiomycetes carry sexual spores externally on club-

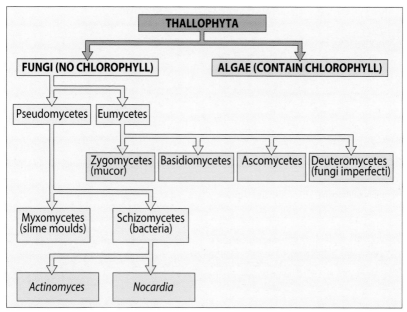

365 Taxonomy of fungi.

shaped cells called basidia. Ascomycetes produce sexual spores within an ascus, and pathogens include *Piedraia hortae*. Most human pathogens are in the taxon Deuteromycotes. They are also called imperfect fungi as they do not reproduce sexually but produce asexual spores on condidia. Pathogenic fungi imperfecti include *Epidermophyton*, *Candida* and *Pityrosporum* spp. A more useful classification is, however, based on disease associations, namely superficial mycoses, subcutaneous mycoses and systemic mycoses (**366**). Although *Actinomyces* spp and *Nocardia* spp are branching bacteria, they are more conveniently covered here.

■ ACTINOMYCETACEAE

These are branching bacteria (**367**) that can be part of the normal flora. The major pathogen is *Actinomyces israelii*, which is Gram positive, non-acid fast

FUNGI AND HUMAN DISEASE	
Superficial mycoses	Dermatophytes (tinea capitis, tinea cruris, tinea pedis, endothrix, ringworm) *Epidermophyton floccosum* *Microsporum audouinii (M. gypseum, M. canis)* *Trichophyton rubrum (T. terrestre, T. mentagrophytes, T. verrucosum, T. violaceum, T. schoenleinii, T. tonsurans)* Pityriasis versicolor – *Malassezia (Pityrosporum) furfur* Black piedra – *Piedraia hortae* Tinea nigra – *Cladosporium werneckii.*
Subcutaneous mycoses	Sporotrichosis – *Sporothrix schenckii* Chromomycosis – *Phialophora verrucosa, Phialophora (Fonsecaea) pedrosisi Cladosporium carrionii.* Mycetoma – *Actinomadura madurae, Nocardia asteroides, Nocardia brasiliensis, Streptomyces somaliensis* Rhinosporidiosis – *Rhinosporidium seeberi* Zygomycosis – *Basidiobalus haptosporus, Conidiobolus coronatus*
Systemic mycoses Primary pathogens	Histoplasmosis – *Histoplasma capsulatum* Coccidiomycosis – *Coccidiodes immitis* Blastomycosis – *Blastomyces dermatitidis* Paracoccidiomycosis – *Paracoccidioides brasiliensis* Cryptococcosis – *Cryptococcus neoformans*
Opportunistic pathogens	*Aspergillus fumigatus* *Candida albicans* *Pneumocystis carinii* *Mucor* spp

366 Fungi and human disease.

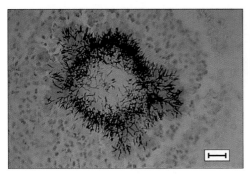

367 Gram-positive *Actinomyces israelii* pus. A Gram film of pus from a patient with abdominal actinomycosis. Branching Gram-positive *Actinomyces israelii* is visible. *(bar = 10 μm)*

and anaerobic or microaerophilic. It produces abscesses in the jaw, chest or abdomen, and is also associated with infections of plastic intrauterine contraceptive devices. Diagnosis is by Gram film of the pus, which may contain sulfur granules (**368**), and culture in liquid or solid media. On solid media, it produces white-gray colonies with an irregular surface resembling the surface of a tooth (**369**). Management is to drain the abscess and treat with penicillin.

■ NOCARDIACEAE
These too are filamentous Gram-positive (**370**) but partially acid-fast bacteria, which, unlike *A. israelii*, also produce bacillary and coccoid forms. *Nocardia asteroides* is found world-wide and causes deep abscesses. *Nocardia brazilensis* and *N. caviae* are a cause of mycetoma (Madura foot). On blood agar, *N. asteroides* produces colonies with an irregular surface.

■ SUPERFICIAL MYCOSES
The dermatophytes are a group of fungi (**371**) that can utilize keratin as a source of nutrition. In the tissues, they are present as hyphae or may divide

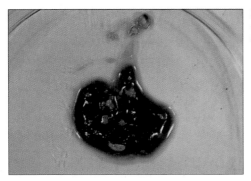

368 Actinomycosis. Sulfur granules from a case of abdominal actinomycosis.

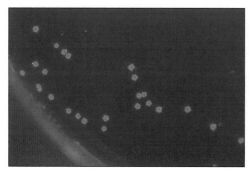

369 *Actinomyces israelii* colonies.
Colonies of *Actinomyces israelii* on
blood agar. These had been
incubated at 37°C under
microaerophilic conditions for
4 days. Note the irregularly shaped
(dentate) colonies.

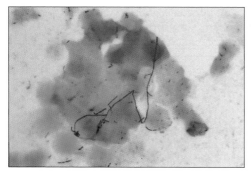

**370 Gram-positive *Nocardia
asteroides* pus.** A Gram stain of pus
containing *N. asteroides*.

THE DERMATOPHYTES		
Anthropophilic	**Zoophilic**	**Geophilic**
Epidermophyton floccosum	*Microsporum canis*	*Microsporum fulvum*
Microsporum audouinii	*M. distortum*	*M. gypseum*
M. ferrugineum	*M. equinum*	*Trichophyton ajelloi*
M. rivalieri	*M. nanum*	*T. terrestre*
Trichophyton concentricum	*M. persicolor*	
T. gourvilii	*Trichophyton equinum*	
T. interdigitale	*T. erinacei*	
T. megninii	*T. gallinae*	
T. rubrum	*T. mentagrophytes*	
T. schoenleinii	*T. quinckeanum*	
T. soudanense	*T. simii*	
T. tonsurans	*T. verrucosum*	
T. violaceum		
T. yaoundii		

371 The dermatophytes.

into arthrospores. On solid culture medium (e.g. Sabouraud's dextrose agar), they produce fluffy or powdery colonies (**372–374**) and their characteristic macro- or microconidia, which permit assignment to species. Biochemical properties are less frequently used for this. *Epidermophyton* spp have rough-walled, pyriform macroconidia (**375**), *Microsporum* spp rough-walled, fusiform macroconidia (**376**) and *Trichophyton* spp smooth-walled, cylindrical macroconidia.

The production of macroconidia by *Trichophyton* spp is poor even when cultured on Sabouraud's malt agar. The diagnostic feature of *T. mentagrophytes* in particular is the production of spiral hyphae (**377**). Infections are termed ringworm or tinea, followed by the site. Thus, tinea capitis is scalp ringworm, tinea corporis body ringworm (**378**), tinea cruris groin ringworm, tinea pedis foot ringworm or athlete's foot, tinea manum hand ringworm, tinea barbae

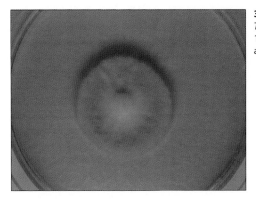

372 *Trichophyton rubrum* culture. *Trichophyton rubrum* cultured for 10 days on Sabouraud's dextrose agar.

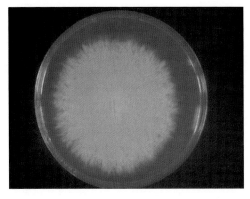

373 *Microsporum gypseum* culture. *Microsporum gypseum* cultured for 10 days on Sabouraud's dextrose agar.

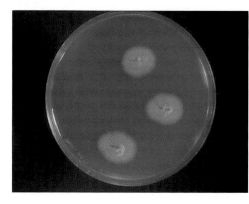

374 *Epidermophyton floccosum* culture. *Epidermophyton floccosum* cultured for 10 days on Sabouraud's dextrose agar.

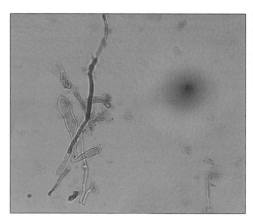

375 *Epidermophyton floccosum* culture. Lactophenol cotton blue-stained preparation of *E. floccosum* cultured on Sabouraud's agar showing the typical pyriform macroconidia.

ringworm of the facial hairs and tinea unguium ringworm of the nails (**379**). Tinea imbricata is caused by *T. concentricum* and is characterized by concentric rings on the skin (**380**). Dermatophytes may also invade hairs; when present on the outside surface, the infection is termed ectothrix, when inside endothrix (**381**). Zoophilic dermatophytes tend to produce a much more florid tissue response and may cause a kerion (**382**).

Diagnosis is by taking skin or nail scrapes or hair samples and placing them in potassium hydroxide (30%) on microscope slides. The slide is then examined for fungal hyphae and arthrospores (**383**). Some dermatophyte lesions (e.g. caused by *M. audouinii, M. canis* or *T. schoenleinii*) fluoresce when exposed to long-wave ultraviolet light (365 nm: Wood's lamp). For precise diagnosis, samples are cultured at room temperature (or better still at 26–28°C) for up to 2 weeks on Sabouraud's dextrose agar.

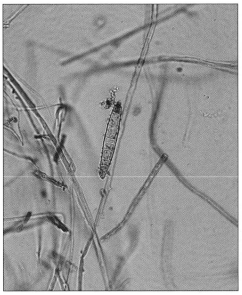

376 *Microsporum canis* culture.
Lactophenol cotton blue-stained
preparation of *M. canis* cultured on
Sabouraud's agar showing the
rough-walled macroconidia.

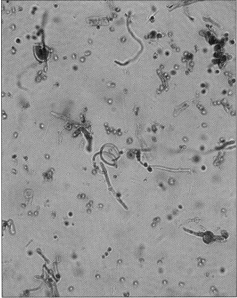

377 *Trichophyton mentagrophytes* culture.
Lactophenol cotton blue-stained
preparation of *T. mentagrophytes*
cultured on Sabouraud's agar
showing spiral hyphae (arrow).

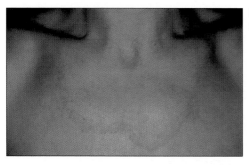

378 Tinea corporis. A case of ringworm (tinea corporis).

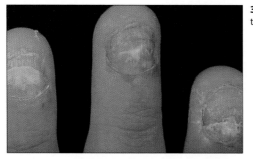

379 Tinea unguium. A case of tinea unguium.

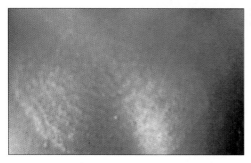

380 Tinea imbricata. A case of tinea imbricata caused by *Trichophyton concentricum*.

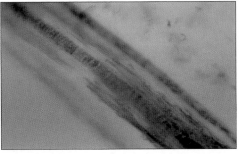

381 Endothrix showing fungal hyphae inside a hair shaft.

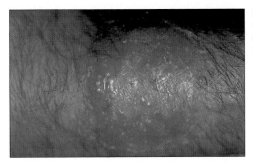

382 A kerion, which is an excessively florid reaction to a zoophilic dermatophyte (*Microsporum canis*).

383 Potassium hydroxide technique showing fungal hyphae. A potassium hydroxide-treated skin scraping showing fungal hyphae and arthrospores.

A small portion of the colony is placed on a microscope slide and spread in lactophenol cotton blue solution. This allows microscopic visualization of the spore arrangements (**375–377**). Treatment, if needed, is with oral griseofulvin.

■ SUBCUTANEOUS MYCOSES

These infections are caused by a variety of fungi and even bacteria but tend to be found in tropical or subtropical regions. The fungi are mostly present in soil and are introduced into the subepidermal tissues by trauma.

Mycetoma

This presents as a destructive localized lesion, most often on the feet (**384**) or hands, with discharging sinuses. Actinomycetoma is caused by bacteria such as *Actinomadura madurae* and *N. asteroides*. Eumycetomata are caused by fungi such as *Madurella mycetomatis*, *Acremonium*, *Aspergillus* and *Fusarium* (**385**) spp. Diagnosis is by microscopic examination of sinus fluid or skin scrapings (potassium hydroxide), but the examination of a biopsy and culture (3–4 weeks) on Sabouraud's agar (without cycloheximide) provides the definitive diagnosis. Treatment involves surgery and appropriate antifungal or antibacterial drugs.

Chromomycosis

This disease is characterized by the appearance of warty nodules and occurs in Africa and Latin America. Pathogens include *Phialophora (Fonsecea) pedrosi*, *P. verrucosa* and *Cladesporium carrionii*.

Sporotrichosis

This is the one subcutaneous mycosis that can occur, albeit rarely, in temperate countries. The causative agent is *Sporothrix schenckii*, which is a

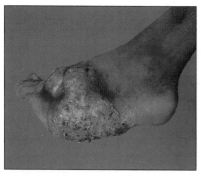

384 Mycetoma of the foot caused by
***Fusarium* spp.**

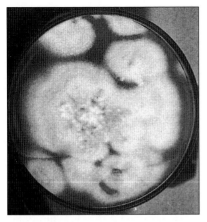

385 *Fusarium* **spp growing on Sabouraud's dextrose agar.**

dimorphic fungus. In human tissues, it is present as the yeast form. It begins as a nodular lesion that may ulcerate. Secondary nodules arise along the lymphatic vessels draining the primary lesion (**386**).

■ SYSTEMIC MYCOSES

Most of these infections result from the inhalation of fungal spores, although *Candida albicans* can be acquired from the gastrointestinal tract or via intravascular lines. Several of the infections, such as histoplasmosis and paracoccidiamycosis, are limited to certain geographical regions where climatic conditions are optimal for their growth. Some affect previously fit individuals, but many are opportunistic pathogens.

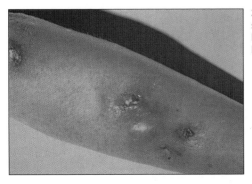

386 Sporotrichosis. A case of sporotrichosis showing secondary lesions along the distribution of the lymphatics.

Aspergillosis

Aspergillus fumigatus, A. flava and *A. niger* are the major pathogens. They are predominantly opportunistic pathogens. They can colonize pre-existing lung cavities to cause an aspergilloma (**387**) or may invade lung tissue and elsewhere when the patient is immunocompromised. They are ubiquitous in the environment. Increases in the infection rate in, for example, bone marrow transplant units have recently been associated with building, excavation or refurbishment in the vicinity of the hospital. *Aspergillus fumigatus* produces smokey green colonies with a velvety texture (**388**), and the conidia produce a columnar mass in the axis of the stalk of the conidiophore (**389**).

Blastomycosis

This infection was thought to be restricted to North America, but cases have been reported from Africa and Asia. *Blastomyces dermatitidis* is a dimorphic fungus the source of which is unknown. Primary lesions occur in the lung, but patients usually present with skin lesions.

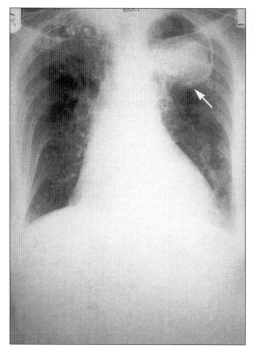

387 Chest X-ray showing an aspergilloma. A chest radiograph showing a lung cavity containing an aspergilloma (arrow).

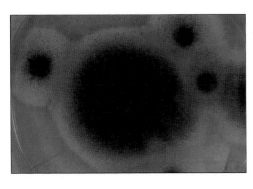

388 *Aspergillus fumigatus* culture.
Aspergillus fumigatus growing on
Sabouraud's dextrose agar.

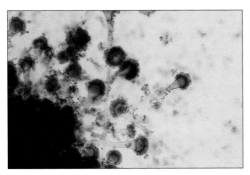

389 *Aspergillus fumigatus* culture.
Lactophenol cotton blue-stained
preparation of *Aspergillus fumigatus*
cultured on Sabouraud's agar
showing a conidiophore and
microconidia.

Candidosis

The major pathogen is *Candida albicans*, but C. *parapsilosis* and C. *tropicalis* may also cause disease. *Candida albicans* can cause superficial as well as systemic infection, but the latter only occurs in immunocompromised individuals. *Candida albicans* is part of the normal flora of the intestine. Superficial infections include oral (**390**) and vaginal thrush, infections of moist skin such as intertrigo (**391**) and those of nails. Disseminated infection can occur in any part of the body. Premature neonates, in particular, are prone to developing urinary tract infection, which ascends to produce a fungal mass in the kidney (**392**). In tissues it is invading, the fungus produces pseudohyphae (**393**).

On a Gram film, large, Gram-positive pleomorphic blastospores are visible (**394**). *Candida* spp grow well on Sabouraud's (**395**) or blood agar. To differentiate C. *albicans* from other species, the yeast is incubated at 37°C in serum, C. *albicans* producing a germ tube (**396**). Nystatin is used for topical therapy and amphotericin B (liposomal or in combination with 5-flucytosine), fluconazole or caspofungin for systemic infection.

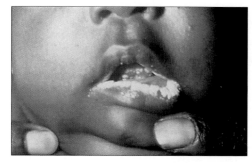

390 *Candida albicans* on oral mucosa. Oral thrush showing a white patch of *C. albicans* on the oral mucosa. Removal of the lesion revealed an inflamed area beneath it.

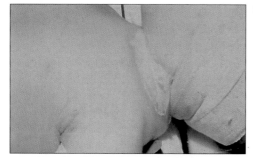

391 Intertrigo.

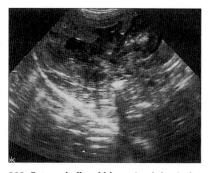

392 Fungus ball on kidney. An abdominal ultrasound of a neonate's kidney showing a fungus ball in the renal calyx. *Candida albicans* was obtained on urine culture.

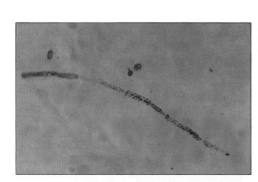

393 *Candida albicans* pus. A Gram-stained preparation of pus from a skin abscess caused by *C. albicans* showing pseudohyphae.

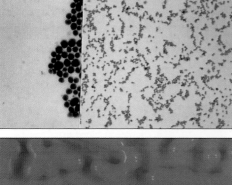

394 *Candida albicans* film compared with *Staphylococcus aureus*. A Gram-stained film of *C. albicans* (left) compared with *S. aureus* (right). *Candida albicans* blastospores are two or three times larger than *S. aureus* cocci.

395 *Candida albicans* culture. *Candida albicans* growing on Sabouraud's dextrose agar.

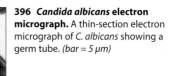

396 *Candida albicans* electron micrograph. A thin-section electron micrograph of *C. albicans* showing a germ tube. *(bar = 5 μm)*

Coccidioidomycosis

The fungus *Coccidiodes immitis* is endemic in dry desert regions of southwestern USA, Mexico and Central America, and is present in soil. Infection is primarily in the lungs, but dissemination can occur.

Cryptococcosis

Cryptococcus neoformans in a dimorphic yeast that is usually associated with opportunistic infection but may also be a primary pathogen. At ambient temperatures it produces hyphae, but at body temperature it is a yeast. It gains access through the lungs but is rapidly disseminated to the central nervous system to cause cryptococcal meningitis. It grows well on Sabouraud's or blood agar (**397**), where it produces mucoid colonies. The mucoid character is imparted by a thick polysaccharide capsule (**398**), which can be seen using India ink stain, either directly on CSF (**399**) or from colonies. A latex particle agglutination test is also available for rapid diagnosis. Treatment is as for disseminated candidosis.

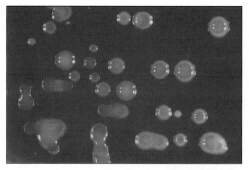

397 *Cryptococcus neoformans* culture. Mucoid *C. neoformans* growing on blood agar. The glistening surface of the colony is caused by the profuse polysaccharide capsule produced by the yeast form.

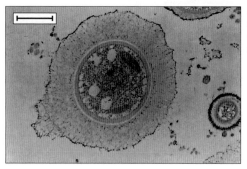

398 *Cryptococcus neoformans* electron micrograph. Thin-section electron micrograph of *C. neoformans* stained by ruthenium red to demonstrate the capsule. *(bar = 5 μm)*

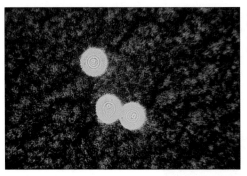

399 Cerebrospinal fluid in cryptococcal meningitis. India ink stain of CSF from a patient with cryptococcal meningitis.

Histoplasmosis

Histoplasma capsulatum causes an acute or chronic pulmonary infection that rarely disseminates. It is found in soil containing bird droppings and, in particular, causes infection in Mississippi and surrounding US states.

Paracoccidioidomycosis

Paracoccidiodes brasiliensis causes oral and pulmonary infection (granulomas). It is restricted to South and Central America.

Zygomycosis (phycomycosis, mucormycosis)

This is a rapidly evolving infection seen in immunocompromised patients. Pulmonary infection is the hallmark of immunocompromise resulting from cytotoxic drug therapy, gastric disease of malnutrition and rhinocerebral infection of diabetes mellitus. Pathogens include *Mucor pusillus* (**400**), *Absidia corymbifera* and *Fusarium* spp.

Pneumocystis carinii

There is some controversy over the kingdom to which this respiratory tract pathogen belongs. It was, on the basis of morphology and antimicrobial susceptibility, originally classified as a protozoan. Recent analysis of gene sequences encoding its 18S ribosomal RNA, however, place it much closer to fungi such as *Candida* and *Saccharomyces* spp. Furthermore, its dehydrofolate reductase (which is inhibited by trimethoprim) and thymidylate synthetase genes are not linked, whereas in protozoa they are encoded on a single gene. Unfortunately, *P. carinii* has not been grown in artificial culture. In immuno-competent individuals, infection is asymptomatic. In those who are immuno-compromised (by AIDS, cytotoxic drugs or even malnutrition), it causes pneumonia. Most evidence suggests that a large number of individuals are exposed at an early age and that the cysts remain in the lungs until immunity is impaired, when they reactivate.

Diagnosis is by the examination of broncho-alveolar lavage by methenamine silver or immunofluorescence (**401**). Lung biopsy may also be of value, when trophozoites and cysts can be demonstrated by electron microscopy (**402**) or silver impregnation stains (**403**). The polymerase chain reaction detection of *P. carinii* genome has recently been used to demon-

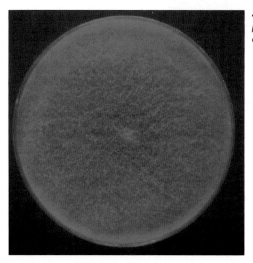

400 *Mucor pusillus* culture. *Mucor pusillus* growing on Sabouraud's dextrose agar.

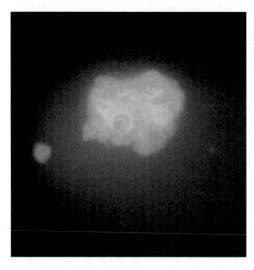

401 *Pneumocystis carinii* by immunofluorescence. *Pneumocystis carinii* demonstrated in a broncho-alveolar lavage by immunofluorescence.

strate the organism in nasopharyngeal aspirates, broncho-alveolar lavage or lung tissue. Treatment is with high-dose co-trimoxazole, dapsone or pentamidine, co-trimoxazole also being used for prophylaxis in the immuno-compromised individual.

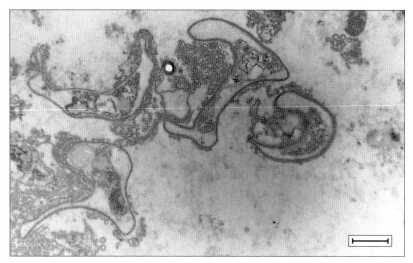

402 *Pneumocystis carinii* electron micrograph of the lungs. Thin-section electron micrograph of the lung showing cysts of *P. carinii. (bar = 5 µm)*

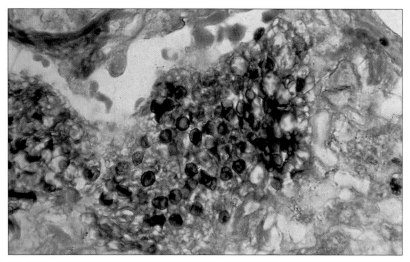

403 *Pneumocystis carinii* cysts. Silver impregnation of a stain of the lung showing cysts of *P. carinii.*

Chapter 7

MEDICALLY IMPORTANT PARASITES

This chapter covers the protozoa (unicellular parasites) and helminths (multicellular parasites) that are encountered in medical microbiology.

■ PROTOZOA

Many different protozoa can be found in the animate and inanimate environment; some (e.g. *Entamoeba coli, Endolimax nana*) are even commensals of man. Only a small number of protozoa are pathogenic for man (**404**). The classification of protozoa is by appearance and biological properties, although a clinically more useful classification is to divide them into mucosal pathogens and tissue and bloodstream pathogens (**405**).

Mucosal Pathogens
Microsporidia
Microsporidia, in particular *Enterocytozoon bieneusii*, can cause diarrhea in immunocompromised patients, particularly those with AIDS. In such patients, it may also cause conjunctivitis. The definitive diagnosis is by demonstrating the organism in biopsy samples of the upper or lower intestine (**406**). They may also be demonstrated by trichrome stain of the feces. Treatment is with co-trimoxazole or albendazole, but relapse is frequent.

Entamoeba histolytica
This ameba has cysts that are difficult to differentiate from the non-pathogenic *Ent. dispar* on stool microscopy. It causes amebic dysentery and can invade beyond the large intestine to cause liver abscesses. It is spread feco-orally by the ingestion of food or water contaminated by cysts (**407**). Specific diagnosis can be by the examination of fresh stools looking for trophozoites containing ingested erythrocytes (**408**). Trophozoites may also be seen in samples scraped from colonic ulcers or even on histological examination of biopsy samples (**409**). Treatment is with metronidazole.

Giardia intestinalis (lamblia)
This is a ubiquitous protozoan parasite with flagellae and a characteristic pear-shaped outline (**410**). It is spread feco-orally and can survive in water

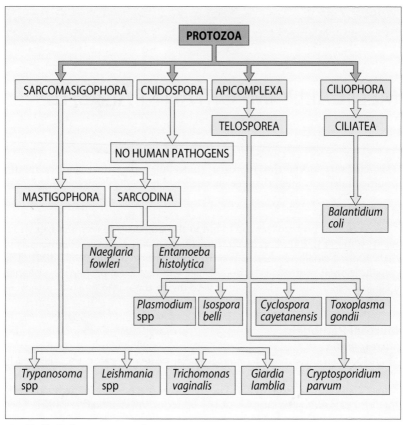

404 Medically important parasites.

for long periods. It is excreted as cysts, which are the infective form (**411**). Giardia infects the proximal small intestine, causing diarrheal disease. Not all infected patients are symptomatic, but infection may also be chronic. Diagnosis is by the examination of stools (at least three samples) for cysts or the examination of duodenal juice (collected by gastroscopy or string) for trophozoites. Treatment is with metronidazole.

Trichomonas vaginalis
This flagellate protozoan parasite can reach a length of 30 μm but is most often in the range 5–15 μm (**412**). As its name implies, it causes vaginitis, with vaginal discharge as the most common presenting feature. The discharge is profuse and can result in perineal inflammation.

PATHOGENIC PROTOZOA	
Mucosal pathogens	**Blood and tissue pathogens**
Enterocytozoon bieneusi – diarrheal disease *Entamoeba histolytica* – dysentery *Giardia lamblia (intestinalis)* – diarrheal disease *Trichomonas vaginalis* – vaginitis *Isospora belli* – diarrheal disease *Cryptosporidium parvum* – diarrheal disease *Cyclospora cayetanensis* – diarrheal disease *Balantidium coli* – dysentery	*Entamoeba histolytica* – liver abscess *Naegleria fowleri* – meningitis *Trypanosoma brucei* – sleeping sickness *T. cruzi* – Chaga's disease *Leishmania donovani* – kala-azar *L. tropica* – oriental sore
	P. falciparum – malignant tertian malaria *P. ovale* – ovale tertian malaria *P. malariae* – quartan malaria
	P. vivax – benign tertian malaria
	Toxoplasma gondii – encephalomyelitis, retinitis

405 Pathogenic protozoa.

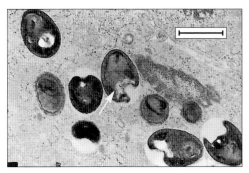

406 *Enterocytozoon bieneusii* electron micrograph. Thin-section electron micrograph of duodenal enterocytes infected with *Enterocytozoon bieneusii* (microsporidiosis). The spirally coiled polar filament (arrow) used for impaling the cell to be infected has been cut in section. *(bar = 100 nm)*

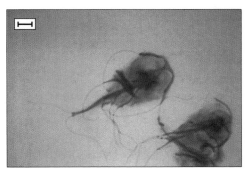

407 *Entamoeba histolytica* cysts and *E. coli*. Iodine-stained wet preparation of stool showing cysts of *E. histolytica* (arrow) and the non-pathogenic *E. coli*. *(bar = 10 µm)*

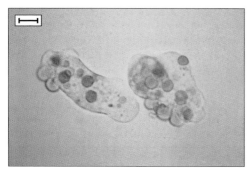

408 *Entamoeba histolytica* trophozoites. Trophozoites of *E. histolytica* that have engulfed erythrocytes. This is pathognomonic of *E. histolytica. (bar = 10 μm)*

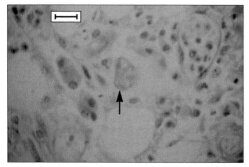

409 *Entamoeba histolytica* found at biopsy. Section of a rectal biopsy stained by hematoxylin and eosin. The section shows an amebic ulcer with an infiltrate of inflammatory cells and *E. histolytica* (arrow). *(bar = 30 μm)*

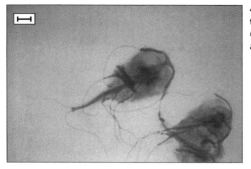

410 *Giardia intestinalis (lamblia)* trophozoites. Trophozoites of *G. intestinalis (lamblia).* The flagella are clearly visible. *(bar = 5 μm)*

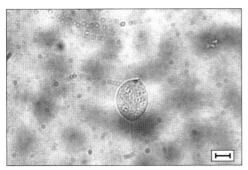

411 *Giardia intestinalis (lamblia)* cysts. Cysts of *G. intestinalis (lamblia)* in feces, viewed by Normarski phase-contrast microscopy. *(bar = 5 μm)*

412 *Trichomonas vaginalis.* Wet preparation of *T. vaginalis* by phase-contrast microscopy. The flagellum that imparts motility is visible. *(bar = 5 μm)*

On colposcopy, the vaginal mucosa is inflamed with punctate lesions. There may also be dysuria and frequency. Infection in males is normally asymptomatic but may rarely cause prostatitis or epididymitis. Diagnosis is by the examination of vaginal discharge by phase-contrast microscopy. Treatment is with metronidazole.

Isospora belli
This is usually an asymptomatic infection but may cause severe diarrheal disease in immunocompromised patients, particularly those with AIDS. It is spread feco-orally, the infective form being the oocyst (approximately 30 × 12 μm), which contains two sporocysts (**413**). The oocyst is immature when excreted and matures in the stool to become infective. Diagnosis is by modified Ziehl–Neelsen or safranin methylene blue (**414**) stains of fecal smears. Co-trimoxazole is the treatment of choice.

Cryptosporidium spp
This small coccidian parasite is a major cause of diarrheal disease in children (2–19% of cases) and a life-threatening pathogen in the immunocompromised host. It is spread feco-orally, and the first reported cases were zoonotic,

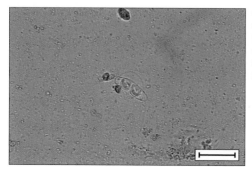

413 *Isospora belli* **oocyst and sporocysts.** Iodine-stained wet preparation of feces showing an oocyst of *I. belli*. The two sporocysts are visible inside the oocysts. *(bar = 20 μm)*

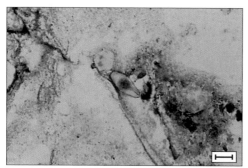

414 *Isospora belli* **oocyst and sporocyst.** An oocyst of *I. belli* stained by safranin methylene blue. The immature sporocyst has retained the safranin (pink), and the cyst wall the methylene blue. *(bar = 10 μm)*

although person-to-person spread is at least as important. This genus of small (4–10 μm) protozoa has recently undergone significant reclassification. *Cryptosporidium hominis* is the major human pathogen, but C. *parvum*, which has microscopically indistinguishable occysts, is the major zoonotic pathogen. Other zoonotic cryptosporidia include C. *canis*, C. *felis*, C. *meleagridis* and C. *muris*.

The oocyst is the infective form (**415**), which is fully infective when excreted and is excreted in large quantities. The oocyst is small (4–5 μm), its thick wall rendering it resistant to many disinfectants. As a result, large water-borne epidemics of diarrheal disease (up to 250 000 patients) have occurred in the USA and UK. The oocyst contains four sporozoites that attach to and penetrate the enterocytes. They develop to form trophozoites, which are described as being intra-enterocytic but extracytoplasmic (**416**) as they are kept from the main part of the enterocyte by a so-called feeder organelle. How they produce diarrhea is unclear. Diagnosis is by the examination of fecal smears by modified Ziehl–Neelson, safranin methylene blue (**417**) or auramine phenol (**418**) stains. Immunofluorescent antigen test and enzyme-linked immunosorbent assay tests are also available for the

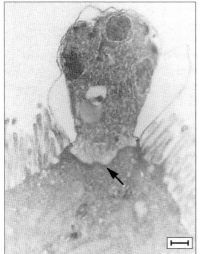

415 *Cryptosporidium parvum* **oocyst electron micrograph.** Negative-stain electron micrograph of an oocyst of *C. parvum*. *(bar = 1 μm)*

416 *Cryptosporidium parvum* **trophozoite found at biopsy.** Thin-section electron micrograph of a duodenal biopsy from a patient with cryptosporidiosis. A trophozoite of *C. parvum* is within the enterocyte but separated from the rest of the cytoplasm by the so-called feeder organelle (arrow). *(bar = 5 μm)*

detection of antigen or of serological response. The newly developed agent nitazoxanide appears to be effective therapeutically.

Cyclospora cayetanensis

This recently described protozoon is a cause of prolonged diarrheal disease. It is spread feco-orally, and water-borne outbreaks have occurred in developing countries. The infective form is the thick-walled oocyst, which is up to $8\,\mu$m in diameter (**419**). Diagnosis is by the microscopic examination of suitably strained fecal smears (**420**). The optimal method is by safranin methylene blue microwave-enhanced staining. Treatment is with co-trimoxazole.

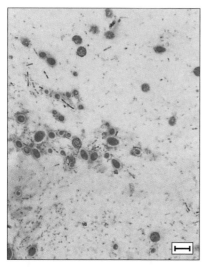

417 *Cryptosporidium parvum* oocysts. A smear of feces stained by safranin methylene blue. The *C. parvum* oocysts stain pink, whereas all other components of the feces stain blue. *(bar = 10 µm)*

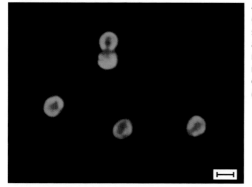

418 Fluorescent microscopy of *Cryptosporidium parvum*. A fecal smear stained by auramine phenol and viewed by fluorescence microscopy. The *C. parvum* oocysts retain auramine phenol, which causes them to fluoresce. *(bar = 5 µm)*

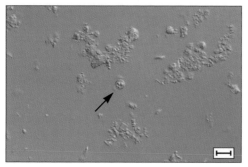

419 *Cyclospora cayetanensis* cysts. A wet preparation of feces containing cysts of *C. cayetanensis* (arrow) viewed by Normarski phase-contrast microscopy. *(bar = 5 µm)*

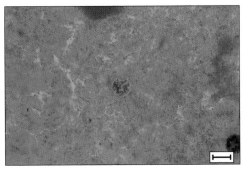

420 *Cyclospora cayetanensis.*
Feces containing *C. cayetanensis*
stained by safranin methylene blue.
(bar = 5 μm)

Balantidium coli

This is the only ciliate to infect man (**421**). It is a rare cause of diarrheal disease. Treatment is with oxytetracycline.

Blood and Tissue Pathogens
Naegleria fowlerii

This is an ambeboflagellate that is in the ameboid form in tissue. It is a rare cause of meningitis and occurs when soil contaminates swimming pools. Cases have been described in individuals swimming in the Roman baths in Bath, UK (warm water being insufflated through the nose). Diagnosis is by the microscopic examination of CSF (where it produces a purulent meningitis). Treatment is with amphotericin B, which might be potentiated by tetracyclines.

Trypanosoma spp

Two distinct forms of disease resulting from trypanosomes occur in man. African sleeping sickness is caused by *Trypanosoma brucei* (*gambiense* or

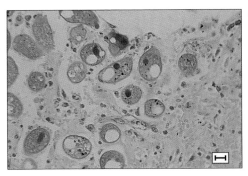

**421 *Balantidium coli* found at
biopsy.** A rectal biopsy showing
infection with *B. coli. (bar = 10 μm)*

rhodesiense). It is transmitted by the bite of the tsetse fly (most frequently *Glossina palpalis* for *T.b. gambiense* and *G. morsitans* for *T.b. rhodesiense*). The East African variety (*T. rhodesiense*) is more virulent but both can lead to meningoencephalitis. The reservoir for *T.b. rhodesiense* is game or domestic cattle; no animal reservoir for *T.b. gambiense* has been identified. Diagnosis is by the identification of trypomastigotes in blood films (**422**). Treatment is with suramin, melarsoprol or pentamidine.

Trypanosoma cruzi is spread via the feces of the reduviid bug (*Panstrongylus megistus*). The trypanosome develops in the hindgut of the reduviid bug, which defecates when biting man. The *T. cruzi* is then introduced into the tissue, producing a chagoma (Romaña's sign, **423**). It spreads via the bloodstream to the liver and spleen, where it may be eliminated. If not, it develops intracellularly (as an amastigote) in cardiac muscle and other tissues. Infection occurs in the Americas, south of the Tropic of Cancer, but is most common in Brazil. Animal reservoirs are cats, dogs and even armadillos. Diagnosis is by demonstration of the amastigote in tissues, and an

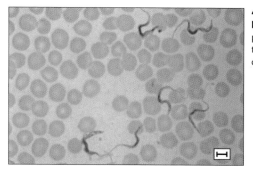

422 *Trypanosoma brucei* **found in blood film.** A blood film from a patient with sleeping sickness. The trypomastigotes of *T. brucei* are clearly visible. *(bar = 5 μm)*

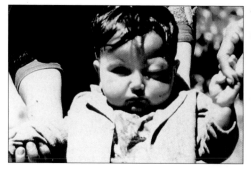

423 A child infected with *Trypanosoma cruzi* **showing Romaña's sign.**

IgM response can be measured. Treatment is with the nitrofurfurylidine derivative Nifurtimox.

Leishmania spp

Oriental sore (**424**) is caused by *L. tropica* and is transmitted by phlebotomine flies (sandflies). It occurs in the Southern and Eastern mediterranean regions, in southern CIS (Armenia, Azerbaijan), Afghanistan and India. Man is the reservoir. Diagnosis is primarily clinical but can also be by the demonstration of amastigotes in monocytic inflammatory cells in the lesion or by culture. Treatment is with pentestam.

Muco-cutaneous leishmaniasis results from *L. brasiliensis* and is endemic in South America, where it is called espundia. Forest rodents and dogs are the reservoirs, the infection being spread by sandflies.

Visceral leishmaniasis is caused by *L. donovani* and is also known as kala-azar. It occurs in many parts of Africa and Asia, and even in southern Europe. Transmission is by plebotomine flies, and the reservoir appears to be dogs. It produces fever, malaise, anemia and hepatosplenomegaly. Diagnosis is by demonstrating the organism in macrophages (**425**) obtained by splenic, bone marrow or hepatic puncture. Treatment is with pentestam.

Plasmodium spp

These protozoa have a complex life cycle in the mosquito and in man. They grow in the anopheline mosquito's intestine, sporozoites being transferred

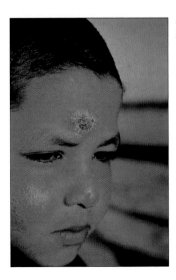

424 A child with oriental sore caused by *Leishmania tropica.*

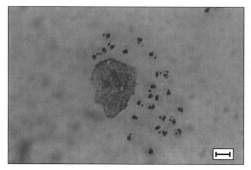

425 Macrophage containing amastigotes. A bone marrow aspirate stained by Giemsa from a child with kala-azar. A macrophage containing numerous amastigotes is visible. *(bar = 10 μm)*

from the female mosquito to man when she next feeds. In man, there are erythrocytic and extraerythrocytic phases. *Plasmodium falciparum* causes malignant falciparum malaria after an incubation period of 8–11 days. Fever occurs every 36–48 h. An untreated primary attack lasts 2–3 weeks, but infection can persist for 6–11 months. The major problems are of cerebral malaria (**426**) and anemia.

Plasmodium vivax causes vivax or benign tertian malaria after an incubation period of 10–17 days. Fever occurs every 48 h, and an untreated primary attack lasts 3–8 weeks or more, although infection can last for 5–7 years. Anemia is the major complication, and mortality is low.

Plasmodium malariae causes quartan malaria after an incubation period of 18–40 days. Fever occurs every 72 h. An untreated primary attack lasts 3–24 weeks, but infection persists for over 20 years with recrudescences. Proteinuria and even frank nephrotic syndrome can be a complication.

Plasmodium ovale causes ovale malaria after an incubation period of 10–17 days. Fever occurs every 48 h. An untreated primary attack lasts 2–3 weeks, but infection persists for up to 12 months. It is usually a mild disease.

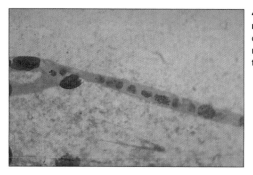

426 Cerebral vessel in cerebral malaria. A cerebral vessel from a child who had died from cerebral malaria. Erythrocytes are adherent to the capillary endothelium.

Diagnosis is by the examination of thick and thin blood films stained by Leishman's or Field's stains (**427–430**). Treatment and prophylaxis depends upon the region where the infection occurs since resistance to chloroquine is increasing in prevalence. Therapeutic options include quinine, artemether, fansidar or halofantrine. Prophylactic drugs include chloroquine, proguanil and mefloquine.

Toxoplasma gondii

This coccidian parasite is found world-wide, its definitive host being the cat. The cat persistently excretes a large number of oocysts in the feces; following maturation, these can infect other species, including man. There are two forms of trophozoites: tachyzoites (**431**), which are rapidly growing, and bradyzoites, which grow very slowly and form cysts. Man may also become infected by eating undercooked meat containing bradyzoites. Infection is asymptomatic in over 50% of cases. When clinically apparent, it causes a glandular fever-like illness and more rarely encephalomyelitis. In immuno-compromised patients, it is more likely to produce encephalomyelitis. *Toxoplasma gondii* can also cross the placenta to infect the fetus. The major problem in the child is chorioretinitis and subsequent blindness. This may develop in up to 60% of those infected in utero, but only a minority of infections present at birth. Cerebral damage with intracerebral calcification (**432**) and microcephaly (**433**) can also occur.

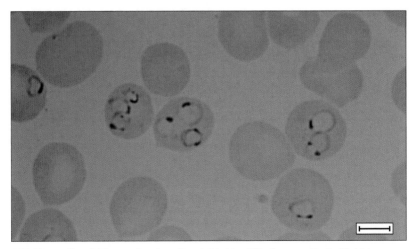

427 *Plasmodium falciparum* **trophozoites.** A thin blood film from a patient with falciparum malaria. Ring forms of the trophozoites of *P. falciparum* are present. *(bar = 5 μm) (Copyright Liverpool School of Tropical Medicine)*

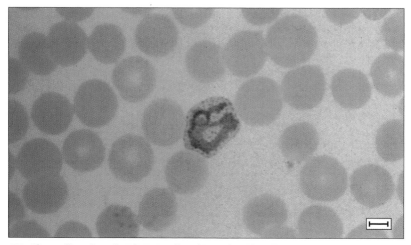

428 *Plasmodium vivax* ring-form trophozoites. A thin blood film from a patient with benign tertian malaria. Both the large ameboid (center) and ring-form trophozoites of *P. vivax* are visible. *(bar = 5 μm) (Copyright Liverpool School of Tropical Medicine)*

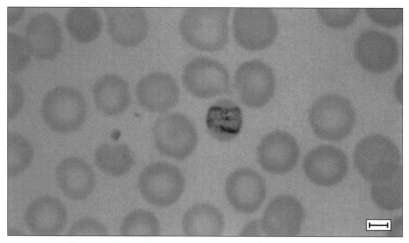

429 Intra-erythrocytic *Plasmodium malariae*. A thin blood film from a patient with quartan malaria. An intra-erythrocytic band form of *P. malariae* is visible. *(bar = 5 μm) (Copyright Liverpool School of Tropical Medicine)*

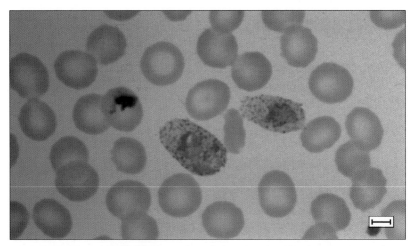

430 Erythrocytes infected with *Plasmodium ovale*. A thin blood film from a patient with ovale malaria. The infected erythrocytes are oval in shape and contain Schüffner's dots and trophozoites of *P. ovale. (bar = 5 μm) (Copyright Liverpool School of Tropical Medicine)*

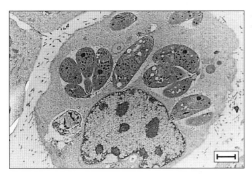

431 *Toxoplasma gondii* tachyzoites. A thin-section electron micrograph of *T. gondii* tachyzoites. *(bar = 5 μm)*

Diagnosis is usually serological (IgM or rising titres), but genome amplification by the polymerase chain reaction is also available. Treatment is with pyrimethamine sulfadoxine.

■ MULTICELLULAR PARASITES

The multicellular parasites are subdivided into Platyhelminthes (flat worms), which contain two classes parasitic on man (Cestodes and Trematodes), and the Aschelminthes, of which the class Nematoda contains human pathogens (**434**).

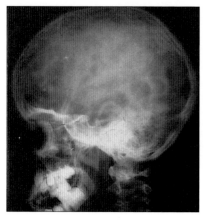

432 Congenital toxoplasmosis. An X-ray of the skull of a child with congenital toxoplasmosis showing intracerebral calcification.

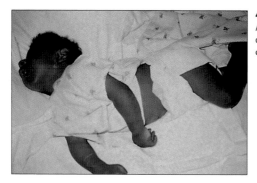

433 Congenital toxoplasmosis. A child with microcephaly and opisthotonos resulting from congenital toxoplasmosis.

Trematodes

Trematodes or flukes have a complex life cycle involving an intermediate host that is a mollusk (usually a snail). The adult develops in man, who excretes ova in which a larva develops. The larva or miracidium infects the mollusk. In the mollusk, the trematode goes through a series of generations, finally liberating more larvae, this time called cercariae. These then infect man by penetrating the skin (e.g. *Schistosoma* spp), by being eaten in a second intermediate host such as fish (e.g *Clonorchis sinensis*) or by attaching to vegetable matter such as watercress that is then eaten (e.g. *Fasciola hepatica*).

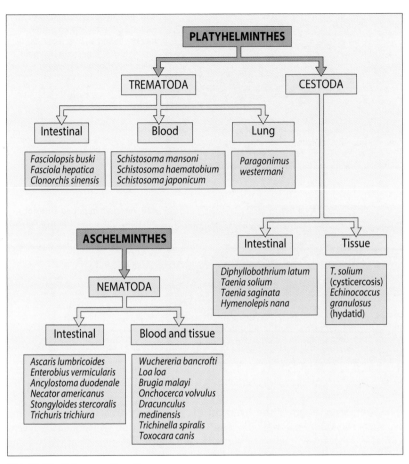

434 Multicellular parasites of man.

Intestinal flukes

Fasciolopsis buski is the giant intestinal fluke (2.0–7.5 cm long) that is found in the Far East. Infection is acquired by eating contaminated water vegetables (e.g. bamboo shoots, water chestnut). Heavy infestation (> 500 worms) results in a disease characterized by yellow, greasy (from malabsorption) stools with vitamin deficiency and hypoalbuminemia. Diagnosis is by the demonstration of ova in the feces (**435**). Treatment is with praziquantel.

Fasciola hepatica (**436**) is the sheep liver fluke and is found in Europe, Latin America and many other areas. The infection is passed to man by the ingestion of watercress to which herbivores, especially sheep, have access.

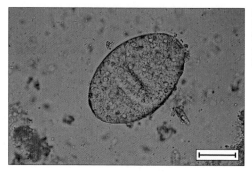

435 *Fasciolopsis buski* ovum. An iodine-stained wet preparation of feces showing an ovum of *F. buski*. *(bar = 40 μm) (Copyright Liverpool School of Tropical Medicine)*

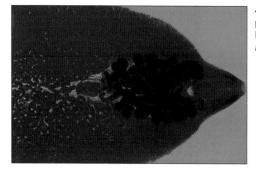

436 *Fasciola hepatica* anterior portion. The anterior portion of the liver fluke, *F. hepatica. (Copyright Liverpool School of Tropical Medicine)*

The metacercaria enter the liver not via the biliary tree but by burrowing through the duodenal wall. Because of this, infection is frequently symptomatic, with fever, chills and signs of cholangitis. Diagnosis is by detecting ova in the stools. Treatment is with praziquantel.

Blood flukes

Schistosoma mansoni is present in Africa, Arabia and Madagascar, and is thought to have been transported to the West Indies and South America via the slave trade. *Schistosoma japonicum* is found in the Far East, and *S. haematobium* has spread from the Nile Valley throughout Africa and to Cyprus, Portugal and the Middle East. Schistosomes, unlike other trematodes, are not hermaphrodites. Miracidia hatch from eggs, are excreted in the stools (*S. mansoni*, *S. japonicum*) or urine (*S. haematobium*) and infect fresh water snails, where they reproduce to release cercaria. The cercaria penetrate intact skin and enter the circulation. *Schistosoma mansoni* lives in the branches of the inferior mesenteric vein (draining the lower colon), *S. japonicum* in the superior mesenteric vein (small intestine) and

S. haematobium in the vesical, uterine and prostatic plexuses. Adult males and females (**437**) mate in the respective veins, eggs being deposited there. They penetrate into the intestine or bladder and are thence excreted. Disease results from the intense inflammation induced by this process. In addition, the initial penetration by the cercaria can cause an intense skin rash and fever (Katayama fever), which can progress to transverse myelitis. Infection is acquired by bathing or paddling in shallow water containing the host snails.

Diagnosis is made by demonstrating eggs in the feces, urine or tissues. *Schistosoma mansoni* has ovoid eggs (150 × 60 μm) with a lateral spine near one pole (**438**), *S. japonicum* is smaller (60 × 50 μm) with a small lateral spine (**439**), and *S. haematobium* a terminal spine (**440**).

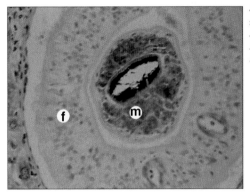

437 *Schistosoma mansoni* in liver section. A section of liver showing adult male (**m**) and female (**f**) *S. mansoni* mating. *(Copyright Liverpool School of Tropical Medicine)*

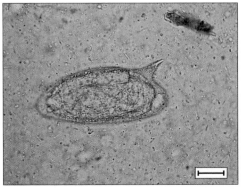

438 *Schistosoma mansoni* ovum. An iodine-stained, wet preparation of feces showing an ovum of *S. mansoni* with a well-demarcated lateral spine. *(bar = 20 μm) (Copyright Liverpool School of Tropical Medicine)*

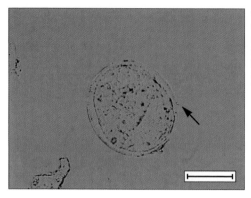

439 *Schistosoma japonicum* ovum. An iodine-stained, wet preparation of feces showing an ovum of *S. japonicum* with a small spine (arrow). *(bar = 20 μm) (Copyright Liverpool School of Tropical Medicine)*

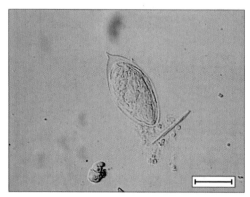

440 *Schistosoma haematobium* ovum. An iodine-stained sample of urine showing an ovum of *S. haematobium* with a terminal spine. *(bar = 50 μm) (Copyright Liverpool School of Tropical Medicine)*

Cestodes

The cestodes are tapeworms that are acquired by the ingestion of improperly cooked fish (*Diphyllobothrium latum*), beef (*Taenia saginata*) or pork (*T. solium*) containing larvae. The beef and pork tapeworms can achieve lengths of 25 m (**441**), infection usually being noticed only when segments are excreted in the feces. Treatment is with niclosamide or praziquantel. If the eggs of *T. solium* (excreted in human feces) are ingested, the larvae invade the intestinal wall, enter the bloodstream and lodge in various tissues, including muscle, brain and retina. Here they grow to produce cysts, which, if in vital areas, lead to cysticercosis. In the brain, for example, they may lead to focal fits, a focal neurological deficit, hydrocephalus or chronic meningitis. Diagnosis is by X-ray (**442**) and the demonstration of cysticerci in the tissues. Treatment is with praziquantel (except for intraocular disease), with dexamethasone to suppress inflammation around the dying cysts.

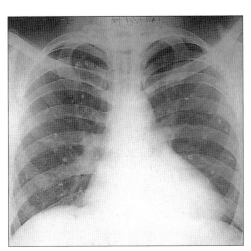

441 Beef tapeworm. A beef tapeworm wrapped around the hands of its host. *(Copyright Liverpool School of Tropical Medicine)*

442 Chest X-ray showing calcified cysts. A chest X-ray showing numerous calcified cysticerci.

The dog tapeworm (*Echinococcus granulosus*) is found particularly in sheep-rearing areas (e.g. New Zealand, Australia, the Balkans, South America). Ingestion of the eggs leads to hydatid disease in man. The larvae penetrate the intestinal mucosae and lodge principally in the liver or lungs. The embryo produces a cyst that continues to grow and may achieve a volume of several litres (**443**). The cyst contains protoscolices, daughter cysts and amorphous debris– 'hydatid sand' (**444**). Cysts are usually first noticed on radiological examination (**445**). Careful aspiration of the cyst will allow demonstration of the hydatid sand. Serological diagnosis is also available. Treatment is surgical removal and, when inoperable, mebendazole.

Nematodes
Nematodes are non-segmented round worms, most of which have a free-living stage.

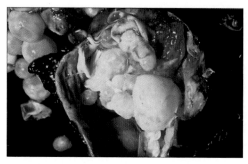

443 Lung showing hydatid cysts. A lung showing several hydatid cysts. *(Copyright Liverpool School of Tropical Medicine)*

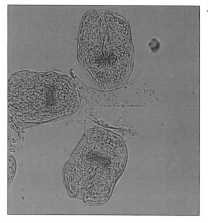

444 Hydatid sand.

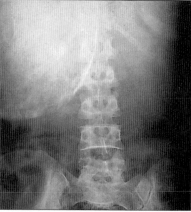

445 Hydatid cysts on liver. An X-ray showing large hydatid cysts on the liver.

Intestinal Worms

Ascaris lumbricoides is a large (20–35 cm) intestinal worm (**446**). Infection is acquired via the ingestion of mature embryonated eggs (**447**). The eggs are excreted in the feces (it was estimated in 1947 that 18 000 tons of *Ascaris* eggs were produced per annum in China). The eggs hatch in the duodenum, the larvae penetrating the intestinal wall, entering the blood or lymphatics and passing to the liver. They then pass to the pulmonary circulation, break into the alveoli, ascend to the pharynx and descend the esophagus to the intestine. There they mate and release eggs (around 200 000 per day). The infection is usually asymptomatic, except during the migratory phase, when asthmatic disease may occur or worms may take a wrong turn and emerge through the nose or mouth. Heavy intestinal infestation may cause obstruction or failure to thrive. Ascaris is found world-wide, especially in areas of poor sanitation. Diagnosis is by the detection of eggs in the feces (**447**). Treatment is with mebendazole.

Enterobius vermicularis, the threadworm, is a common infection of children world-wide. The adult worm resides in the cecum and adjoining areas.

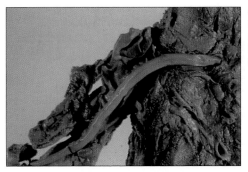

446 *Ascaris lumbricoides* in a renal vein. The roundworm *A. lumbricoides*. It escaped from the intestine following a knife wound and lodged in the renal vein.

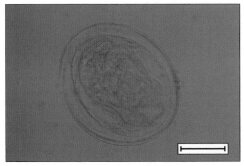

447 *Ascaris lumbricoides* ovum. An ovum of *A. lumbricoides* in feces. The larva is visible inside the egg. *(bar = 20 µm) (Copyright Liverpool School of Tropical Medicine)*

Gravid females (**448**) migrate to the anus, where they deposit eggs on the anal verge (**449**). This is intensely irritant and causes the child to scratch, the eggs then being transferred to fingers and thence to the mouth to autoinfect or infect others. The clinical features vary according to the amount of irritation, but it often interferes with sleep since the worms come out at night. They may also migrate to the vagina, causing vulvovaginitis. Diagnosis is by the cellophane tape method. The tape is applied to the anal verge early in the morning and picks up eggs. The tape is then stuck to a microscope slide and examined using a ×10 objective, under which the eggs are clearly visible (**449**). Treatment is with mebendazole or pyrantel pamote. The whole family must be treated.

The hookworms *Ancylostoma duodenale* and *Necator americanus* both infect man by penetrating the intact skin, usually that of the feet. Man appears to be the only host of *A. duodenale*, but rabbits, lambs and calves can be experimentally infected with *N. americanus*. *Ancylostoma duodenale* is found in Europe, South America, India, China and the Pacific Islands. *Necator americanus* is found in sub-Saharan Africa and was probably taken

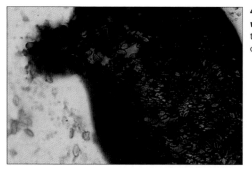

448 Female *Enterobius vermicularis*. A gravid female threadworm, *E. vermicularis*, full of ova.

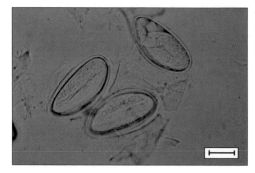

449 *Enterobius vermicularis* ova. Eggs of *E. vermicularis*. (bar = 20 µm)

to America (North and South) by the slave trade. Hookworm eggs (**450**) are excreted in feces and hatch preferably on moist sandy soil to produce larvae (rhabditiform). They then molt to become filariform or infective larvae, which wait until a suitable bit of human skin is available. They are carried to the lungs by the bloodstream, where they burrow into the alveoli. They then ascend to the pharynx and descend the esophagus to the small intestine. Here they attach to the wall by means of teeth or cutting plates. Penetration of the skin is accompanied by pruritis (ground itch), and when they enter the lung they may cause pneumonitis. Once in the intestine, they may cause abdominal pain, but with persistent heavy infestation the major problem is one of severe iron deficiency anemia. Diagnosis is by demonstrating eggs in the feces (**450**). Treatment is with mebendazole.

Stongyloides stercoralis has a similar geographic distribution to the hookworm. Cats and dogs may also be infected. Under optimal environmental conditions (moist and warm), the free-living rhabditiform larvae can go through several generations. They eventually transform into the infective filariform larvae, which congregate together (**451**) and enter man by penetrating the skin. Thereafter, the path is similar to that of the hookworm. Unlike the hookworm, *S. stercoralis* is usually excreted as rhabditiform larvae rather than eggs, and these larvae may transform to filariform infective larvae in the intestine, setting up repeated cycles of infection in the same host. Infection thus persists for decades. There are, for example, a number

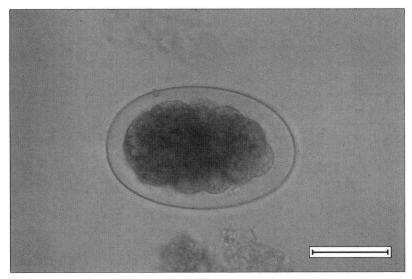

450 *Ancylostoma duodenale* ovum. An ovum of the hookworm, *A. duodenale*, in feces. *(bar = 20 µm)*

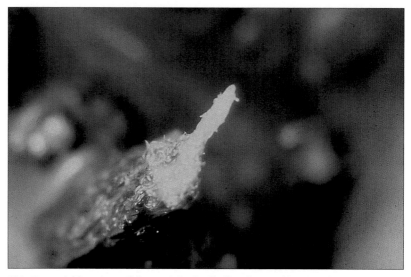

451 *Strongyloides stercoralis* **larvae.** Infective filariform larvae of *S. stercoralis* on soil ready to penetrate the exposed skin of the unwary. *(Copyright Dr R. Ashford)*

of British soldiers who were kept in Japanese prisoner of war camps who are still infected 50 years later. Patients may develop pulmonary symptoms as the worms pass through the lung, or malabsorption from heavy intestinal parasitism. Worms occasionally lose their way and produce cutaneous larva migrans (**452**). When infection is very heavy or the immune system is suppressed, a life-threatening hyperinfection of disseminated strongyloidiasis occurs, with Gram-negative septicemia and penetration of the worms into the heart, liver, lungs, kidneys and central nervous system. Diagnosis is by the demonstration of larvae in the stools (**453**) or by duodenal aspiration. Serological tests are available in specialized centers. Thiabendazole is the drug of choice but is compromised by a high incidence of side-effects and incomplete efficacy.

Trichuris trichiura, the whip worm (**454**), has a world-wide distribution and is acquired feco-orally. It mostly produces asymptomatic infection but may rarely give rise to abdominal distension, bloody mucoid diarrhea, weight loss and anemia if the infection is heavy. Diagnosis is by demonstrating the characteristic barrel-shaped eggs in the stools (**455**). Treatment, if necessary, is with mebendazole.

Blood and Tissue Nematodes

The filaria (*Wuchereria bancrofti, Loa loa, Onchocerca volvulus, Brugia malayi*) are widely distributed in the tropics and subtropics. They all have an

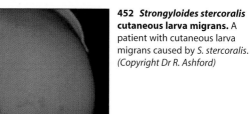

452 *Strongyloides stercoralis* **cutaneous larva migrans.** A patient with cutaneous larva migrans caused by *S. stercoralis*. *(Copyright Dr R. Ashford)*

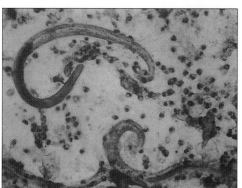

453 *Strongyloides stercoralis* **larvae.** Rhabditiform larvae of *S. stercoralis* in feces. *(Copyright Dr C. Parry)*

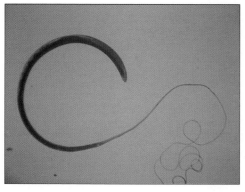

454 *Trichuris trichiura.* The whipworm *T. trichiura. (Copyright Liverpool School of Tropical Medicine)*

insect (mosquito, mango fly, black-fly) as an intermediate host and are deposited on humans when they are bitten. The filaria produce lymphatic blockage leading to lymphedema (**456**), cutaneous larva migrans or ocular damage depending on the particular worm. It has recently been discovered that the filarial worms all have an obligate intracellular bacterial symbiont called *Wolbachia*. If the bacteria are killed by, for example, tetracycline, the worm dies. Thus, new antibacterial therapies are now available to treat filariasis.

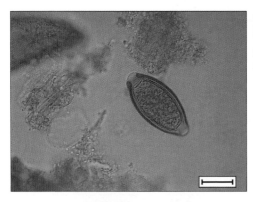

455 *Trichuris trichiura* wet preparation. An ovum of *T. trichiura* in a wet preparation of feces stained with iodine.
(bar = 20 μm)

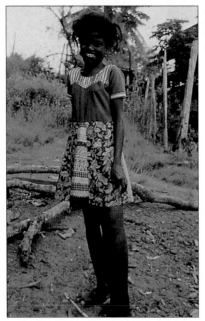

456 Elephantiasis caused by *Wuchereria bancrofti*. An African child with elephantiasis (lymphedema) caused by *W. bancrofti*.
(Copyright Liverpool School of Tropical Medicine)

The guinea worm (*Dracunculus medinensis*) is found in Africa, the Nile Valley and Asia as far east as central India and Pakistan. The adult female can grow to 1.5 m (**457**), but the male is far less impressive, at a mere 2 cm long. The gravid female is present in the subcutaneous tissue and at the head end produces a skin blister (**458**); this, when put in warm water, bursts, releasing a large number of larvae. These are then ingested by *Cyclops* spp, where they mature. If the *Cyclops* spp are ingested by humans, the larvae penetrate the intestinal wall, entering deep connective tissue where they mature and mate. The infection becomes apparent when the gravid female emerges (**458**). Treatment is with mebendazole or niridazole. Elimination of the guinea worm is a World Health Organization goal and can be achieved by the proper control of drinking water.

Trichinella spiralis is transmitted to man by the consumption of under-cooked, contaminated pork or other meat. In the intestine, male and female worms mate to produce larvae. These burrow through the intestinal wall to the lymphatics and thence to the bloodstream. They then penetrate the sheaths of striated muscle, where they encyst (**459**). Muscle invasion is characterized by fever, eosinophilia, muscular pain and tenderness,

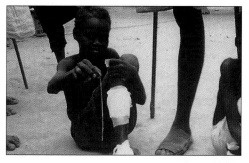

457 *Dracunculus medinensis.* A Sudanese boy displaying the guinea worm (*D. medinensis*) that has been removed from his leg.

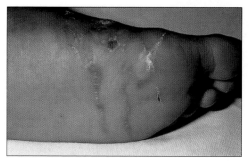

458 *Dracunculus medinensis* blister with larvae. A blister caused by *D. medinensis* on the foot of a Nigerian child. The blister is full of larvae. The worm can be seen winding subcutaneously across the sole of the foot.

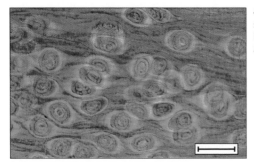

459 Trichinella spiralis larvae. A section of muscle full of *T. spiralis* larvae. *(bar = 10 μm) (Copyright Liverpool School of Tropical Medicine)*

circumorbital edema being a pathogenomic sign. The organism may also invade the brain, causing encephalitis. Diagnosis is by serology or the demonstration of encysted organisms in muscle. Treatment aims primarily to damp down inflammation (dexamethasone). The role of thiabendazole or mebendazole is unclear.

Visceral larva migrans in temperate countries is principally caused by *Toxocara canis* or *T. cati*. As these names imply the adult worms are present in the intestine of dogs and cats (**460**). The ova are excreted in the feces and mature outside the host. Humans (particularly children) become infected by the ingestion of cat or dog feces. In the human intestine, the eggs hatch, penetrate through the intestinal wall and enter the tissue (viscera). Here they encyst. The clinical features can vary from none with eosinophilia to hepatomegaly with eosinophilia, to retinitis (**461**) through to severe pulmonary disease and death. The latter is fortunately very rare. Diagnosis is on clinical grounds. Serology and laparoscopy are adjuncts to diagnosis. Treatment is usually not given, but thiabendazole can be used if necessary.

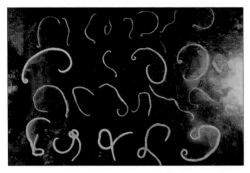

460 Adult *Toxocara canis*. Adult *T. canis* worms from dog feces. *(Copyright Dr R. Ashford)*

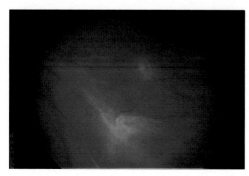

461 *Toxocara canis* **retinitis.**

Chapter 8

MEDICALLY IMPORTANT INSECTS AND OTHER ECTOPARASITES

The phylum arthropoda (Greek, *arthron* = joint, *pous* = foot) contains numerous (over 800 000) genera and species, most of which are not harmful to man. The medically important arthropods fall into six classes (**462**). It is, however, more clinically useful to classify them into agents that directly cause disease (**463**) and those which act as vectors for other diseases (**464**). From these, it can be seen that some arthropods fall into both classes.

■ AGENTS DIRECTLY CAUSING DISEASE
Leeches
Land leeches are found in India, south-east Asia and parts of Oceania and South America. Aquatic leeches have a world-wide distribution. They are annelid worms with specialized chitinous mouthparts and secrete an anti-

THE MEDICALLY IMPORTANT ARTHROPODS	
Insecta or Hexapod	True insects with a head, thorax and abdomen. The only class in which some members possess wings (e.g. flies, fleas, lice, mosquitoes, bugs)
Arachnida	Possess a fused head and thorax (cephalothorax) and abdomen but no feelers or antennae (e.g. ticks, mites, spiders, scorpions)
Crustacea	Possess a head, thorax and abdomen. Distinguished from all other arthropods by having two pairs of antennae (e.g. crabs, lobsters, water fleas)
Chilipoda	Possess a head and a long, dorsoventrally flattened, fused thoraco-abdomen made up of numerous similar segments. Each segment has a pair of walking legs. The first pair of legs is modified to form poison claws (e.g. centipedes)
Diplopoda	Possess a head bearing mouthparts and antennae. The cylindrical thoraco-abdomen is made up of numerous identical segments most of which have a pair of legs. The anterior genital opening differentiates millipedes from centipedes (e.g. millipedes)
Pentastomida	Were previously classified as nematodes, but the larvae of some possess appendages. The pathogens are highly specialized endoparasites of man (e.g. *Armillifer* and the tongue-worm, *Linguatula*)

462 Medically important arthropods.

ARTHROPODS AND OTHER ECTOPARASITES THAT INDUCE DISEASES DIRECTLY BY TRAUMA, POISON OR HYPERSENSITIVITY	
Annelida	Land leeches (e.g. *Haemadipsa* spp)
	Aquatic leeches (e.g. *Limnatis* spp)
Insecta	Myiasis – cutaneous or body cavity maggots (e.g. *Cordylobia anthropophagea*)
	Jiggers (e.g. *Tunga penetrans*)
	Lice (pubic lice, *Phthirus pubis*; head (body) louse, *Pediculus* (corporis) *capitis*)
	Hymenoptera* (e.g. bees, wasps, hornets, ants)
	Fleas* (e.g. *Pulex irritans*)
	Mosquitoes* (e.g. *Aedes* or *Anopheles* spp)
	Midges* (e.g. *Culicoides* spp)
	Tabanidae (e.g. horse-fly: *Tabanus* or *Chrysops* spp)
	Bugs (e.g. bed bugs, *Cimex*; reduviid, *Triatoma* or *Panstrongylus* spp)
Arachnida	Spiders (e.g. black widow, *Lactrodectus mactans* or funnel web, *Atrax robustus*)
	Scorpions (e.g. *Antroctonus crassicauda*)
	Ticks (e.g. *Dermacentor andersoni*)
	Mites (e.g. *Sarcoptes scabiei*; house dust mite*, *Dermatophagoides pteronyssinus*)
Chilipoda	Centipedes (e.g. *Scolopendra* spp)
Diplopoda	Millipedes (e.g. *Rhinocricus*, *Spirobolus* and *Spirastreptus* spp)
Pentastomida	Tongue worm (*Linguatula* spp)

*Some or all of the damage is caused by hypersensitivity.

463 Arthropods and other ectoparasites that induce diseases directly by trauma, poison or hypersensitivity

ARTHROPODS AS VECTORS OF DISEASE		
	Vector	**Diseases**
Insecta	Sandflies (Phlebotominae)	Leishmaniasis, Oroya fever (bartonellosis), phlebovirus
	Mosquitoes (*Aedes, Anopheles, Culex*)	Alphaviruses, flaviviruses, bunyaviruses, malaria, filariasis
	Blackfly (*Simulium*)	Onchocerciasis
	Tabanidae (*Chrysops*)	Loiasis (Calabar swelling)
	Tsetse fly (*Glossina*)	African trypanosomiasis (sleeping sickness)
	Flies	Diarrheal disease, trachoma
	Lice (*Pediculus*)	Typhus, trench fever, relapsing fever
	Bugs (*Cimex*)	? Hepatitis B
	Bugs (*Reduviidae*)	Chagas' disease (South American trypanosomiasis)
	Fleas	Plague (*Yersinia pestis*), typhus
Arachnida	Ticks (*Ixodes, Ornithodoros*)	Lyme disease (*Borrelia burgdorferi*), relapsing fever (*B. hermsi, B. duttoni*), Rickettsiae, flaviviruses, alphaviruses, bunyaviruses, babesiosis
	Mites (*Trombiculidae*)	Scrub typhus
Crustacea	Water flea (*Cyclops*)	Guinea worm (*Dracunculus medinensis*), *Diphyllobothrium latum*
	Crabs, crayfish	*Paragonimus westermani*

464 Arthropods as vectors of disease.

coagulant, hirudin. Land leeches have strong jaws that can penetrate external skin (**465**), whereas aquatic leeches are weaker and attack mucous surfaces. Leeches can cause severe loss of blood; if the leech is pulled off, the jaws may remain in the skin and lead to secondary infection. Leeches can be induced to release themselves by heat (a match or cigarette), hypertonic salt solutions, alcohol or vinegar. Leeches are also used for beneficial purpose, for example for removing subcutaneous collections of blood.

Myiasis

This condition occurs when the larvae of dipterous flies invade the tissues and develop into maggots. This can occur on skin or within body cavities. Some are facultative invaders of pre-existing wounds (e.g. *Lucilla* spp), but some can invade intact skin. The maggot (**466**) of the tumbu fly (*Cordylobia anthropophaga*) develops from eggs deposited in clothing and invades skin to produce a carbuncle-like lesion (**467**). The lesion is less painful than a boil, and close inspection reveals not pus but the respiratory spiracles of the maggot. To remove the maggot from the mature lesion, it should be covered with Vaseline or paraffin oil (**468**) to asphyxiate it. It will then wriggle partly out and can be gently squeezed from its burrow. Prevention is by hanging clothes to dry where the fly cannot reach and carefully ironing the seams of

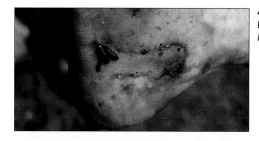

465 Land leeches. Land leeches in Papua New Guinea. *(Copyright Dr R. Ashford)*

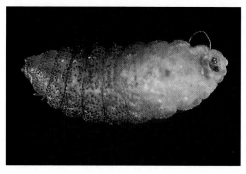

466 *Cordylobia anthropophaga* maggot. The maggot of the tumbu fly (*C. anthropophaga*). *(Copyright Liverpool School of Tropical Medicine)*

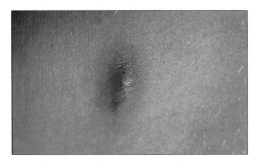

467 *Cordylobia anthropophaga* lesion. A carbuncle-like lesion of the tumbu fly maggot. *(Copyright Liverpool School of Tropical Medicine)*

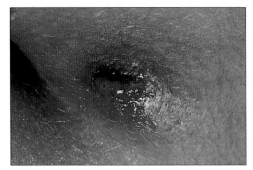

468 *Cordylobia anthropophaga* maggot emerging. The same lesion treated with Vaseline to cause the maggot to emerge. *(Copyright Liverpool School of Tropical Medicine)*

clothing to destroy the eggs. Other maggots, such as *Dermatobia hominis*, have large spines and must be removed surgically. Myiasis of body cavities such as the sinuses or middle ear is caused, for example, by the screw fly (*Chrysomia bezziana*) and is much more damaging, with a measurable mortality (up to 8%). Some maggots (e.g. *Lucilla*) have been used therapeutically to débride wounds.

Jiggers and other Fleas

Jiggers are burrowing fleas (*Tunga penetrans*) that can produce painful and even crippling lesions (**469**). The adults are free-living, but when fertilized the female flea attaches to a suitable host (poultry, pigs, man, other animals) and penetrates cracks or crevices in the skin. Inside the crevice, the gravid female flea grips firmly and swells, often to the size of a pea (**470**). After 8–12 days, the swelling is large enough to cause irritation. Severe inflammation is followed by ulceration and the expulsion of a large number of eggs. Secondary infection and even tetanus may follow. Treatment is by removing the jigger with a sterile needle (without its bursting) and covering the lesion with sterile dressings and antiseptics. Prevention is by wearing an appropriate foot covering, since this flea cannot jump well, and using a 'scorched earth' policy.

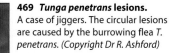

469 *Tunga penetrans* lesions.
A case of jiggers. The circular lesions
are caused by the burrowing flea *T.
penetrans. (Copyright Dr R. Ashford)*

**470 The gravid female *Tunga
penetrans.***

Other fleas produce localized irritation or allergy. The human flea *Pulex
irritans* is diminishing in importance. Most human flea bites are caused by
cat and dog (*Ctenocephalides felis* or *C. canis*) fleas (**471**). The rat flea
(*Xenopsylla cheopis*) is the classic vector of plague (*Yersinia pestis*) and
murine typhus (*Rickettsia mooseri*). This and other fleas may transmit dwarf
tapeworms (*Hymenolepsis* spp), if accidentally ingested. An increasing resistance to DDT is being observed, and malathion may be more effective.

Lice

Three species of lice infest man, namely *Phthirus pubis* (the pubic or crab
louse), *Pediculus corporis* (the body louse) and *Pediculus capitis* (the head
louse). The latter two are in fact very similar, differing only in minor anatomical
details, and are often grouped as *Pediculus humanus.*

Head lice infect the hair-covered areas of the head (**472**). The adults roam
over the scalp. They feed by grasping the skin with a sucking mouth, the
haustellum, and penetrate the skin to draw blood via two stylets. After
fertilization, the female grasps a hair and cements an egg to the shaft, leaving
the characteristic nit (**473**). Nits are deposited at a rate of 7–10 per day, and
the female is reproductively active for about a month. The total cycle from

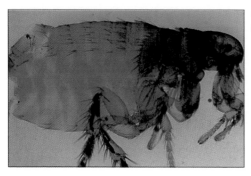

471 *Ctenocephalides canis.* The dog flea.

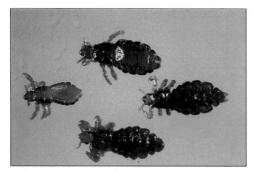

472 *Pediculus capitis.* Head lice.

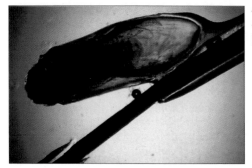

473 Nit with emerging louse.
A nit with a louse about to emerge.
(Copyright Liverpool School of Tropical Medicine)

egg to egg lasts about 16 days. Head lice are spread by close contact and are endemic in many schools. They are not usually vectors of disease and can be managed by removing the nits with a fine comb and treatment with an appropriate insecticide (e.g. malathion). It is not necessary to shave the head.

Body lice flourish under conditions of poor hygiene. They infest areas of the body that are covered by hairs but prefer areas that are also covered by clothes. Body lice are found world-wide but tend to be most prevalent in conditions of relative cold. They are spread by close contact and shared clothes or bedding. The female lays eggs on body hairs but more frequently (70% of the eggs) on fibers in clothes or bedding. They are the sole vector of louse-borne typhus (*Rickettsia prowazeki*), louse-borne relapsing fever (*Borellia recurrentis*) and trench fever (*Bartonella quintana*). Malathion is used to control body lice on man. Lice cannot survive without feeding on man for more than 10 days; thus they do not persist in houses. The nits will survive on clothing for up to 4 weeks. Nits are destroyed by heating at 70°C for 30 min.

Pubic lice (**474**) have crab-like claws on their second and third legs with which they grasp the pubic hairs. They are rather sluggish and are usually confined to the pubic region, although they can infest beards, eyebrows and eyelashes (**475**). *Phthirus pubis* is still killed by DDT. DDT is not, however, active against the nits, and malathion is preferred.

Hymenoptera

There are over 4000 species of stinging bees, wasps and hornets. The direct damage induced by the sting is usually local (redness, pain, swelling) and short-lived. The venom is injected through a barbed sting and contains a variety of biactive amines (e.g. histamine), enzymes (e.g. phospholipase A) and toxic peptides (e.g. mellitin). Death can occur as a result of hypersensitivity (present in 0.5% of the population) to the venom, resulting in anaphylaxis. The most common stings are those of wasps (**476**) and honey bees (*Apis mellifera*). Local treatment involves removal of the sting (as it

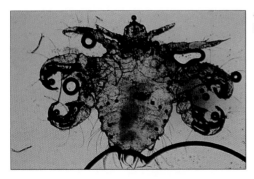

474 *Phthirus pubis.* The crab or pubic louse.

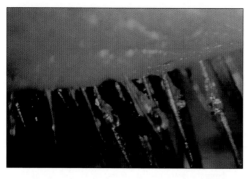

475 Pediculosis. Lice infestation can involve even the eyelashes.

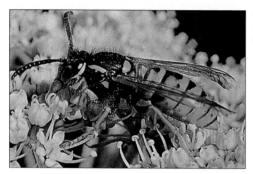

476 The common wasp (*Vespula vulgaris*). *(Copyright Liverpool School of Tropical Medicine)*

continues to inject venom) and perhaps local antiseptics. The management of anaphylaxis requires subcutaneous adrenaline (0.5–1 ml 0.5% solution), maintenance of the airway and urgent hospitalization.

Mosquitoes

There are at least 35 genera of mosquito, found world-wide from above the Arctic circle to well below the equator. The adults of both sexes feed on nectar, but some also suck the blood of a variety of animal and bird species. Hypersensitivity to the saliva of the mosquito results in the appearance of mosquito bites. Female mosquitoes are, however, also important vectors of disease. *Anopheles* spp (**477**) are important biological (i.e. the agent replicates in the mosquito) vectors of malaria, filariasis, alphaviruses (e.g. Venezuelan equine encephalitis), flaviviruses (e.g. St Louis encephalitis) and bunyaviruses (e.g. Tahyna), although they are not the principal vector of the latter three. *Aedes* spp (**478**) also transmit filariasis and are major vectors of alphaviruses (e.g. Chikungunya), flaviviruses (e.g. Dengue and yellow fever) and some bunyaviruses (e.g. Californian encephalitis).

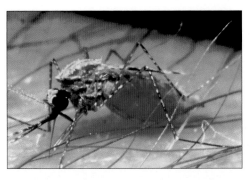

477 Anopheles mosquito. An anopheles mosquito close to the end of a meal. *(Copyright Liverpool School of Tropical Medicine)*

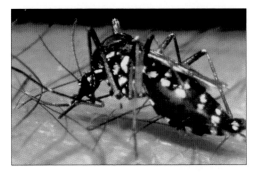

478 *Aedes aegypti*. *Aedes aegypti* feeding. *(Copyright Liverpool School of Tropical Medicine)*

Tabanidae

This family includes several flies that pose a biting nuisance and are the largest blood-sucking flies, with a wingspan of over 6 cm. Only the females bite, and they can take a large blood meal (20–200 mg). In addition, *Chrysops* spp (**479**) are the biological vectors of loaiasis (Calabar swelling caused by *Loa loa*). Other Tabanidae may also be mechanical vectors of anthrax, tularemia and perhaps Lyme disease.

Bugs

Bed bugs have a world-wide distribution. The major parasites of man are *Cimex lectularius* (**480**) and *C. hemipterus* (principally in the tropics). Females lay up to 100 eggs in a life time. These are deposited in cracks and crevices in walls, behind pictures and wallpaper, and in beds and mattresses. The bugs produce irritating bites and may be a vector of hepatitis B virus.

Spiders

There are numerous genera of spiders, most of which cause no harm. Large hairy spiders are usually harmless, relatively small insignificant-looking ones

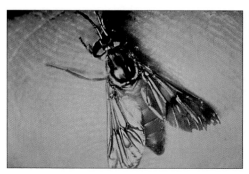

479 Chrysops dimidiata. A mango fly. *(Copyright Liverpool School of Tropical Medicine)*

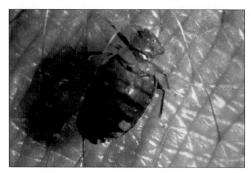

480 Cimex lectularius. A bed bug.

being the most poisonous. In general, the venoms are necrotizing or neutrotoxic. The black widow spider (*Lactrodectus mactans*, **481**) produces a powerful neurotoxin and was responsible for 63 deaths in USA over a 10 year period in the 1950s. The funnel web spiders include *Atrax robustus*, which is found in and around Sydney, Australia.

Scorpions

Scorpions (**482**) are widely distributed in the tropics and subtropics. They deliver venom via a comma-shaped sting at the top of the tail. Following stinging, the mortality rate can be as high as 55%, especially in young children. In Mexico, there is an incidence of death of 84 per 100 000 per year in Colima state. The venoms produce both local necrosis and neurotoxic features.

Mites

Mites and ticks are in the subclass *Acari*, in which there are over 30 000 species. Although there are over 200 families of mites, only a few affect man.

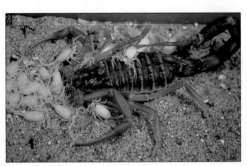

481 *Lactrodectus mactans.* The black widow spider. *(Copyright Liverpool School of Tropical Medicine)*

482 Scorpion. *(Copyright Liverpool School of Tropical Medicine)*

Sarcoptes scabei causes scabies (**483**) and is found world-wide. Its incidence increases greatly in times of war, famine or other disasters. It is spread person to person by close contact in families and can be spread by sexual contact. It is estimated that, in the British Army in the Second World War, as many as 6000 new cases were diagnosed per month. The adult scabies mite (**484**) is a small (250–350 µm) flattened disc with eight, short, squat legs. The fertilized female burrows into the skin for several millimeters to centimeters (never below the stratum corneum). The sites chosen are where the skin is thin and wrinkled, for example the wrists, exterior surfaces of the elbows, axillae, penis, scrotum and under the breasts. As she is burrowing, the female lays 20–30 eggs, which hatch into larvae within 4–5 days. In the burrow, the larvae molt into nymphs and then again to become adult females. The lifespan from egg to egg takes 2–3 weeks. Treatment is of all the family with benzyl benzoate, eurax or gamma benzene hexachloride. Scabies is transmitted only by close contact so there is no absolute need to disinfect the bedding.

Demodex follicularum (follicle mites, **485**) cause no disease apart from perhaps neuroses. They are normal inhabitants of the skin follicles of the eyelids, nose and face.

Dermatophagoides pteronyssinus, the house dust mite (**486**) feeds, as its name implies, on desquamated skin. It can reach very high population

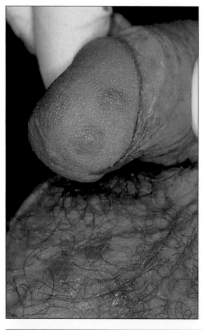

483 Genital scabies. A patient with genital scabies. Each lesion is a burrow containing *Sarcoptes scabiei.*

484 *Sarcoptes scabiei.* The scabies mite (*Sarcoptes scabiei*). *(Copyright Liverpool School of Tropical Medicine)*

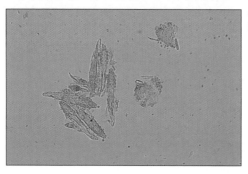

485 *Demodex folliculorum.* The follicle mite.

densities in pillows, mattresses and settees. The feces of the mite are a potent allergen, inducing asthma and allergic rhinitis. Control is by treating infected sites with insecticides and regular vacuum cleaning.

Centipedes
Centipedes (487) also have a world-wide distribution, but it is only the large tropical and subtropical varieties that can inflict harmful bites. The venom, which is delivered by claws adapted from the first pair of legs, produces localized necrotic lesions.

Millipedes
Millipedes (488) differ from centipedes in having a cylindrical body and many more segments and legs (literally a thousand legs). They either secrete or forcibly eject a toxic fluid from specialized glands. It is very irritant to skin, conjunctivae and other mucous membranes.

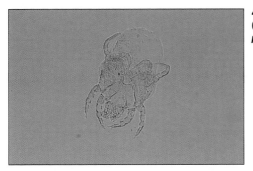

486 The house dust mite (*Dermatophagoides pteronyssinus*).

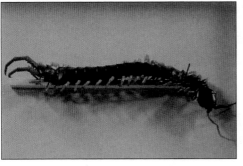

487 Centipede (*Scolopendra* spp).

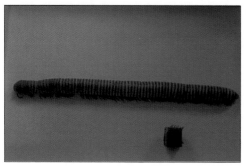

488 Millipede.

Pentastomida

This comprises two genera: *Linguatula* (**489**) and *Armillifer* (**490**). Adult *Linguatula* live in the nasal passages of dogs, wolves and foxes. Man can become infected by the ingestion of either eggs (visceral liguatulosis) or larvae. In the latter, the larvae become established in the nasal passages producing halzoun (hoarseness, dysphagia, dyspnea, vomiting). *Armillifer* is acquired by eating raw python or other snakes or drinking water contaminated by snakes. Disease is usually asymptomatic, although there can be liver damage (**491**).

■ VECTORS OF DISEASE
Phlebotomine sandflies

The sandflies are *Phlebotomus* (**492**) in the Old World and *Lutzomyia* in the New World. Only the females feed on blood. Bites may result in an urticarial reaction, but the flies' most important role is as vectors of cutaneous and visceral Leishmaniasis, Oroya fever (in the Andes) and phleboviruses (sandfly or papatosi fever).

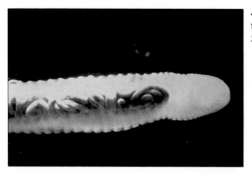

489 *Linguatula serrata.* The tongue worm. *(Copyright Liverpool School of Tropical Medicine)*

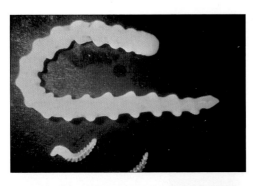

490   *Armillifer armillatus.* *(Copyright Liverpool School of Tropical Medicine)*

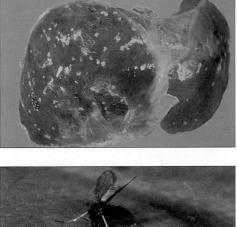

491   Liver granulomas and calcification owing to *Armillifer armillatus.* *(Copyright Liverpool School of Tropical Medicine)*

492   A sandfly (*Phlebotomus papatasi*) feeding. *(Copyright Liverpool School of Tropical Medicine)*

Blackfly
It is the female *Simulium* spp (**493**) that feeds on blood. These transmit the filiarial parasite *Onchocerca vovlulus*, causing onchocerciasis, in both Africa and South and Central America.

Tsetse fly
The tsetse fly or *Glossina* spp (**494**) is confined to tropical Africa. The flies are attracted by bright colors and powerful odors. They produce painful bites. More importantly, they are the vector of sleeping sickness (*Trypanosoma brucei*).

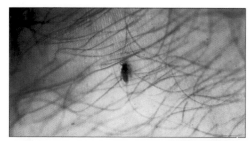

493 A blackfly (*Simulium damnosum*) feeding. *(Copyright Liverpool School of Tropical Medicine)*

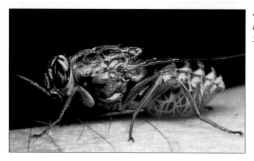

494 A tsetse fly (*Clossina morsitans*). *(Copyright Liverpool School of Tropical Medicine)*

Bluebottle
Bluebottles (**495**), and house flies can act as mechanical vectors of diarrheal pathogens and trachoma (*Chlamydia trachomatis* A–C).

Bugs
Triatomite or reduviid bugs (**496**) defecate as they bite the skin and thus release *Trypanosma cruzi*, which enter the bite. This results in a local chagoma (Romaña's sign) and subsequently Chagas' disease (South American typanosoniasis).

Ticks
All ticks are obligate blood-sucking parasites (**497, 498**). There are two basic forms: soft or argasid ticks and hard or ixoidid ticks. The hard ticks are slow

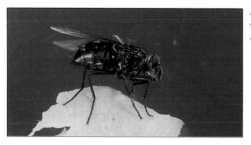

495 A bluebottle (*Calliphora* spp) feeding. *(Copyright Liverpool School of Tropical Medicine)*

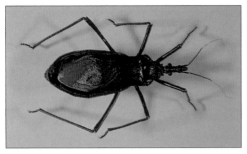

496 A reduviid bug (*Triatoma dimidiata*). *(Copyright Liverpool School of Tropical Medicine)*

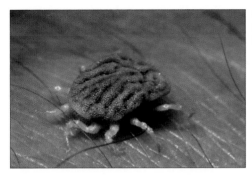

497 A soft tick (*Ornithodorus moubata*) about to feed. *(Copyright Liverpool School of Tropical Medicine)*

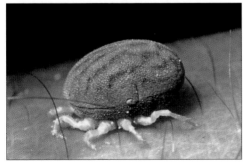

498 *Ornithodorus moubata* engorged with blood. The same tick engorged with blood. *(Copyright Liverpool School of Tropical Medicine)*

feeders and remain attached for days, whereas the soft ticks feed quite often overnight. Most feed on domestic or other animals, feeding on man only by chance. The soft tick of southern Africa (*Ornithodorus moubata*) is the only one to specialize in man and poultry. Soft ticks transmit tick-borne relapsing fever (*Borellia duttoni*, *B. hermsii*, *B. persica*) to man in Africa, Asia America and even Mediterranean Europe. The hard ticks (e.g. *Ixodes ricinus*) transmit Lyme disease (*B. burgdorferi*), ehrlichiosis, rickettsioses (fièvre boutonneuse, Rocky Mountain spotted fever, Siberian tick typhus), babesiosis, flaviviruses (Kyansur Forest and Omsk hemorrhagic fever) and bunyaviruses (Congo-Crimean hemorrhagic fever).

Chapter 9

EMERGING, RE-EMERGING AND ZOONOTIC INFECTIONS

Now is a particularly exciting time for the study of the interactions between microbes and man. Not only do we have new understandings of how bacteria and viruses cause disease, but there has also been a rapid increase in knowledge on the range of microbes pathogenic to man. It is estimated that there are at least 1415 different pathogenic microorganisms that infect man. These comprise 217 different prions and viruses, 538 bacteria, 307 fungi, 66 protozoa and 287 helminths. Of these, 868 (61%) are zoonotic, i.e. transmitted to humans from other animals. A total of 175 (12%) are emerging, i.e. detected in the past 30 years, examples of these being shown in **499**. It is noteworthy that three-quarters of the emerging pathogens are zoonotic. In addition, diseases we thought were contained, such as tuberculosis, and infections thought to be geographically limited, such as West Nile virus, have expanded their operations and re-emerged.

Although reference to zoonoses dates from as early as Biblical times (*Deuteronomy* 14:8), we still do not have an ideal classification system. A recently proposed system is shown in **500**. This is based on the evolutionary origin of zoonoses and leaves room for future additions to the expanding list of zoonotic pathogens. Some recent emerging and re-emerging pathogens are examined below.

PRIONS AND VIRUSES
Variant Creutzfeld–Jakob Disease
In 1985, the first case of 'mad cow' disease (bovine spongiform encephalopathy) was detected and was soon followed by a major epidemic in cattle. Worries that the prion responsible might infect humans were realized when patients with variant Creutzfeld–Jakob disease (vCJD) were described. vCJD differed from classical CJD in that the progression to death was longer, it was occurring in patients under 40 years of age and the histopathological picture was different. On section, the brain showed large plaques of prion protein deposition (**501**) that were reminiscent of those seen in kuru. This led to great public health concerns, but the UK beef industry is now BSE-free, and the number of cases of vCJD remains small, with a decreasing prevalence.

EXAMPLES OF 'NEW' AND EMERGING PATHOGENS OVER THE PAST 30 YEARS

Year	Pathogen	Year	Pathogen	Year	Pathogen
1973	Rotavirus	1983	Human papillomavirus 16	1993	Baylisascaris procyonis
1975	Human parvovirus	1984	Capnocytophaga canimorsus	1993	Simkania negevensis
1975	Tanapoxvirus	1985	Rhodococcus equi	1993	Trophyrema whippelii
1975	Lassa virus	1985	HIV-2	1993	Human granulocytic ehrlichia
1976	Monkeypoxvirus	1985	Birnavirus	1994	Sabia virus
1976	Calicivirus	1985	Vibrio vulnificans	1994	Hendra virus
1976	Cryptosporidium parvum	1985	Chlamydophila pneumoniae	1995	Hepatitis G virus
1977	Clostridium difficile	1986	Strongyloides fullebornii	1995	Human herpes virus 8
1977	Ebola virus	1986	Cyclospora cayetanensis	1996	Whitewater Aroyo virus
1977	Flexal virus	1988	Human herpesvirus 6	1996	Australian bat lyssavirus
1977	Legionella pneumophila	1989	Ehrlichia chaffeensis	1996	Variant CJD
1977	Hepatitis D virus	1989	Hepatitis C virus	1996	Tula virus
1977	Campylobacter jejuni	1989	Human pestivirus	1997	Laguna Negra virus
1980	Enteropathogenic Escherichia coli	1990	Human herpesvirus 7	1997	Andes virus
1980	Astrovirus	1990	Hepatitis E virus	1997	Menangle virus
1980	HTLV-1	1991	Guanarito virus	1997	TTV
1980	Haemophilus ducreyi	1992	Vibrio cholerae 0139	1998	Nipah virus
1982	Escherichia coli O157	1992	Rickettsia felis	1998	Human torovirus
1982	HTLV-2	1992	Enteroaggregative E. coli	1999	SEN virus
1982	Borrelia burgdorferi	1992	Enterocytozoon bieneusii	2001	Human metapneumovirus
1983	HIV-1	1992	Campylobacter upsaliensis	2002	Bermejo virus
1983	Mobiluncus spp	1992	Bartonella henselae	2002	Burkholderia anthina
1983	Helicobacter pylori	1993	Sin nombrevirus	2002	Inquilinus limosus
1983	Adenovirus 40/41	1993	Neisseria weaveri	2003	SARS coronavirus

CJD = Creutzfeldt–Jakob disease. HTLV = human T-cell leukemia/lymphoma virus. TTV = transfusion-transmissible virus.

499 Examples of 'new' and emerging pathogens over the past 30 years.

CLASSIFICATION OF ZOONOSES	
Old zoonoses	Endemic and epidemic human-specific infections with a temporally distant non-human source (e.g. measles, coronaviruses, smallpox)
Recent zoonoses	New or emerging human epidemic or endemic infections with a recent non-human source (e.g. HIV-1 from chimpanzees, HIV-2 from macaques)
Established zoonoses	Infectious diseases with a non-human reservoir host that are occasionally transmitted to humans (e.g. rabies, non-typhoidal salmonellae, *Campylobacter*)
New and emerging zoonoses	Infectious diseases with a non-human reservoir that have only recently spread (or been observed to spread) to humans (e.g. hanta, Ebola, hendra and nipah viruses, *Ehrlichia chaffeensis*)
Parazoonoses	Epidemic or endemic human infectious disease that periodically changes in virulence after an input of genes from non-human pathogens (e.g. antibiotic resistance transferred from animal to human bacteria or genomic reassortment (antigenic shift) in influenza A or rotavirus)

500 Classification of zoonoses.

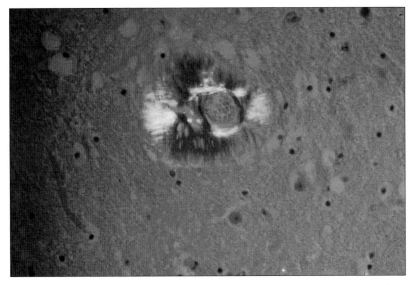

501 Large amyloid plaques of variant Creutzfeld–Jakob disease stained by Congo red.

Hendra, Menangle and Nipah Viruses

These paramyxoviruses have emerged as causes of fatal encephalitis over the past decade. The most recent, Nipah virus (**502**), is persistently excreted by fruit bats of the genus *Pteropus* (**503**). The introduction of large pig-farming operations in Malaysia led to pigs being infected (usually a respiratory infection), pig farmers, farm workers, veterinarians and abattoir workers becoming infected with fatal encephalitis.

Human metapneumovirus

This paramyxovirus is a member of the Pneumovirinae and is related to respiratory syncytial virus (RSV). Like RSV, it causes respiratory tract infections and, in infants, bronchiolitis. It can occasionally be fatal (**504**). Although it was first described in 2001, there is no doubt it has been a cause of infection for a long time.

West Nile Virus

This enveloped RNA virus is part of the Japanese encephalitis subgroup of the genus *Flavivirus* family Flaviviridae. It was first isolated in Uganda in 1937 and was responsible for sporadic and epidemic febrile illnesses in Africa, the Middle East and Asia. In 2000, it emerged in the USA and in 2002 caused a large outbreak of encephalitis with 225 deaths. West Nile virus is usually transmitted between a large number of bird species, especially

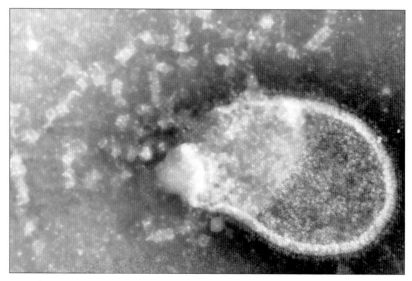

502 Nipah virus.

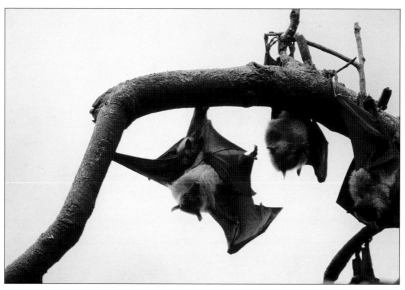

503 The fruit bat *Pteropus vampyrus*, a reservoir of Nipah virus. (Copyright Masahiro Iijiama/ardea.com)

the crow family Corvidae (**505**) by culicine mosquitoes (**506**). Since the same mosquitoes will also bite humans, they may become infected too. The human viremia is low level and transient so human-to-human transmission via mosquitoes is rare, although there have been a number of cases in the USA transmitted by blood transfusion.

Monkeypox

This DNA virus (**507**) causes an illness similar to smallpox but with a lower mortality (approximately 10%). It is zoonotic, and a number of West African mammals appear to be persistently infected, man and monkeys becoming accidentally infected by contact. However, a recent outbreak in Zaire was characterized, unusually, by person-to-person spread. In May 2003, cases of monkeypox were found in the USA. This seems to have been a result of importing, as pets, giant Gambian rats, which infected prairie dogs kept in the same pet shop. Human owners of the prairie dogs were bitten and developed monkeypox.

■ BACTERIA

Two recently described infections are monocytic and granulocytic ehrlichiosis. Monocytic ehrlichiosis is caused by *Ehrlichia chaffeensis*. It is transmitted to humans from its reservoir (deer) by hard ticks (e.g. *Amblyomma* spp). So far, it has been limited to the USA.

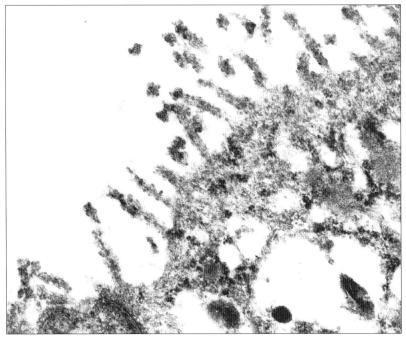

504 Thin-section electron micrograph of a section of lung from a fatal case of infection with human metapneumovirus showing virus budding from pneumocytes.

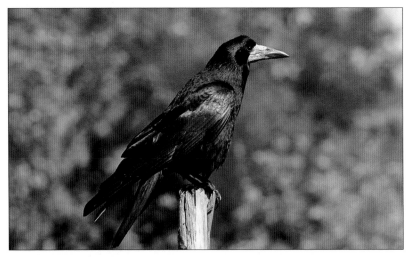

505 Rook (*Corvus frugilegus*), a reservoir host for the West Nile virus. (Copyright J B Bottomley/ardea.com)

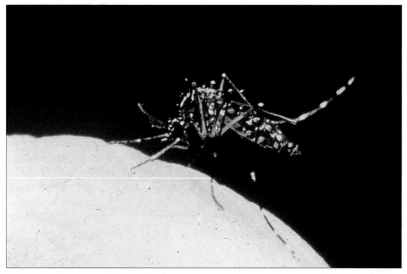

506 Mosquito vector of West Nile virus.

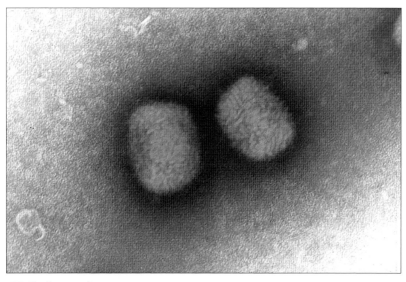

507 Monkeypox virus.

The agent of human granulocytic ehrlichiosis, which was first described in 1993, has been renamed *Anaplasma phagocytophilum*. It is transmitted by ixodid ticks and is unusual in that it replicates inside neutrophils (**508**). It causes an acute febrile illness that can be immunosuppressive and produce an AIDS-like disease.

■ PARASITES

Microsporidia such as *Enterocytozoon bienusii* are important causes of chronic diarrhea in patients with AIDS (**509**).

Filarial worms are transmitted to humans by insects and cause lymphatic blockage leading to elephantiasis (e.g. *Wuchereria bancrofti*) or ocular infections (e.g. *Loa loa*). These worms have as obligate intracellular bacterial symbionts *Wolbachia* spp (**510**). If the bacteria are killed, the worms, both larval and adult forms, die. This opens up the possibility of therapy with antibiotics such as tetracycline.

The fox tapeworm *Echinococcus multilocularis* is endemic in China (**511**). When humans ingest food contaminated with feces containing eggs of *E. multilocularis*, they develop a potentially fatal disease, alveolar echinococcosis (>95% mortality untreated). There is evidence that the prevalence is increasing in Europe and that its geographical distribution has greatly increased into Western Europe.

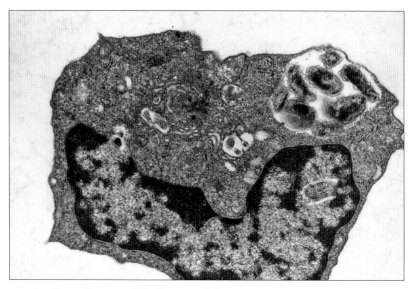

508 *Anaplasma phagocytophilum* in neutrophils.

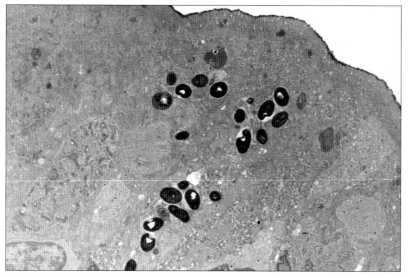

509 Human colonic cells containing the microsporidian parasite *Enterocytozoon bienusi.*

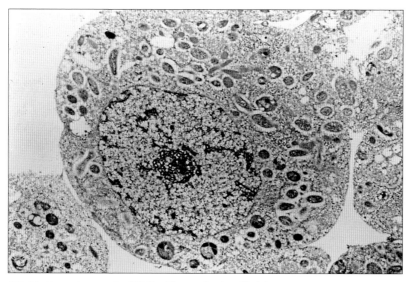

510 Electron micrograph of *Wolbachia* growing in a filarial worm.

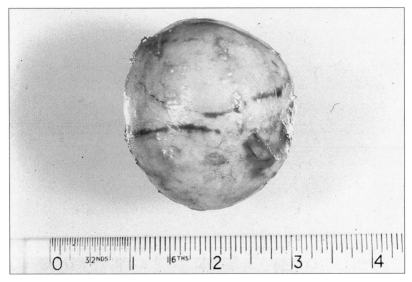

511 Surgically removed cyst of *Echinococcus multilocularis*.

APPENDICES

NERVOUS SYSTEM INFECTIONS			
	Most important	**Less common**	**Tropical or geographically limited**
Encephalo-myelitis	Enteroviruses (including polio) Human herpesviruses (HHV) 1 and 2 Human immunodeficiency virus (HIV) Mumps	HHV-3[a], 4[a] and 5 Influenza A and B[a] Lymphocytic choriomeningitis virus Measles[a] Rubella[b] *Borrelia burgdorferi* *Leptospira* spp *Listeria monocytogenes* *Mycobacterium tuberculosis* *Mycoplasma pneumoniae* *Cryptococcus neoformans* *Naegleria fowleri* *Toxoplasma gondii*	Bunyaviruses Rabies Togaviruses *Borrelia recurrentis* *Brucella* spp *Rickettsia* spp *Trophyrema whippelii* *Histoplasma capsulatum* *Plasmodium falciparum*
Acute meningitis Neonate	HHV-1 and 2 Enteroviruses *Escherichia coli* Group B streptococci *L. monocytogenes*	*Enterobacter* spp *Haemophilus influenzae* b *Klebsiella* spp *Neisseria meningitidis* *Salmonella* spp *Streptococcus pneumoniae* *Candida albicans*	
[a]Infective and post infective-encephalomyelitis. [b]Only post infective or post vaccination.			

Appendix 1 Nervous system infections.

NERVOUS SYSTEM INFECTIONS (*Cont'd*)			
	Most important	**Less common**	**Tropical or geographically limited**
Older individuals	Enteroviruses Mumps *H. influenzae* b *N. meningitidis* *S. pneumoniae*	Adenovirus HIV, HHV-2 Lymphocytic choriomeningitis virus Measles *Borrelia burgdorferi* Enterobacteriaceae *Leptospira* spp *L. monocytogenes* *M. tuberculosis* *Treponema pallidum*	Togaviruses
Chronic meningitis	*M. tuberculosis* *Cryptococcus neoformans*	*Borrelia burgdorferi* *Brucella* spp *Leptospira* spp *L. monocytogenes* *N. meningitidis* *T. pallidum* *C. albicans*	*Francisella tularensis* *Blastomyces dermatitidis* *Coccidoides immitis* *Histoplasma capsulatum*
Intracranial suppuration *Local spread*			
from mucosal surfaces	Polymicrobial: anaerobes, *Streptococcus* spp, Enterobacteriaceae	–	–
by trauma or surgery	Mono- or polymicrobial: *Staphylococcus aureus*, Enterobacteriaceae, *Pseudomonas* spp	–	–
from meningitis	*H. influenzae* b *L. monocytogenes* *Citrobacter diversus*	–	–
Bacteremic spread	Enterobacteriaceae *Salmonella* spp *S. aureus* Viridans streptococci *Candida* and *Aspergillus* spp	*Burkholderia pseudomallei*	–

[a]Infective and post infective-encephalomyelitis. [b]Only post infective or post vaccination.

Appendix 1 Nervous system infections (*cont'd*).

NERVOUS SYSTEM INFECTIONS (*Cont'd*)			
	Most important	**Less common**	**Tropical or geographically limited**
Spinal cord and peripheral nerves *Toxins*	*Clostridium botulinum* *C. tetani* *Corynebacterium diphtheriae*	–	–
Infections			
Cord	Polioviruses 1, 2, 3 *Treponema pallidum*	Enteroviruses (70, 71) Coxsackie A, B *Borrelia burgdorferi* *Brucella* spp	*Schistosoma* spp
Peripheral nerves	Varicella-zoster (HHV-3)	–	*Mycobacterium leprae*
Post infectious or post vaccination			
Guillain–Barré	Epstein–Barr virus and cytomegalovirus (HHV-4, 5), HIV, rubella	*Borrelia burgdorferi* *Campylobacter jejuni* *Salmonella typhi*	Human T-cell lymphotrophic virus I (HTLV-1) *Trophyrema whippelii*

[a]Infective and post infective-encephalomyelitis. [b]Only post infective or post vaccination.

Appendix 1 Nervous system infections (*cont'd*).

HEAD AND NECK INFECTIONS	
Mouth	
Caries	*Streptococcus mutans*
Gingivitis	HHV-1
	Spirochaetes and *Prevotella intermedia* (acute necrotizing ulcerative gingivitis)
Periodontitis	Spirochaetes, *Porphyromonas gingivalis*, *Actinobacillus actinomycetemcomitans*
Thrush	*Candida albicans*
Dental abscess	Polymicrobial; anaerobes
Rhinitis	Adenovirus, coronaviruses, influenza virus, parainfluenza virus, respiratory synctial virus, rhinoviruses
Tonsils and pharynx	Adenoviruses, coronaviruses, enteroviruses, HHV-4, influenza virus, parainfluenza virus, respiratory synctial virus (RSV), *Arcanobacterium haemolyticum*, *Chlamydia pneumoniae*, *Corynebacterium diphtheriae*, *C. ulcerans*, *Mycoplasma pneumoniae*, *Neisseria gonorrhoeae*, *Streptococcus pyogenes* (group A), *C. albicans*
Vincent's angina	*Bacteroides* spp, *Fusobacterium* spp
Peritonsillar abscess	
(Quinsy)	*Sreptococcus pyogenes*, anaerobes
Ludwig's angina	Polymicrobial, anaerobic streptococci, *Bacteroides* spp, *Fusobacterium* spp
Retropharyngeal abscess	Polymicrobial, anaerobes, staphylococci, streptococci
Sinuses and middle ear	
Acute	Respiratory viruses
	Haemophilus influenzae, *Moraxella catarrhalis*, *Staphylococcus aureus*, *Streptococcus pneumoniae*, *Streptococcus pyogenes*
Chronic	Anaerobes, Enterobacteriaceae, *Pseudomonas* spp
Parameningeal structures	
(subdural abscess, epidural abscess)	Polymicrobial anaerobes, Enterobacteriaceae, *Pseudomonas* spp, *Staphylococcus aureus*, streptococci

Appendix 2 Head and neck infections.

RESPIRATORY TRACT INFECTIONS	
Laryngo-tracheobronchitis	Adenovirus, enterovirus, influenza virus, parainfluenza virus, RSV, rhinovirus, *Haemophilus influenzae* (secondary infection), *Staphylococcus aureus, Streptococcus pneumoniae*
Laryngeal papillomata	Human papillomavirus
Epiglottitis	*H. influenzae* b (*S. pneumoniae, S. aureus*; rare)
Bronchiolitis	RSV, adenovirus 7
Whooping cough	*Bordetella pertussis, B. parapertussis*, adenovirus
Community-acquired pneumonia	Adenovirus, influenza virus, measles, parainfluenza virus, RSV, *Chlamydia pneumoniae, C. psittaci, Fusobacterium necrophorum, H. influenzae, Legionella pneumophila, Moraxella catarrhalis, Mycobacterium tuberculosis, Mycoplasma pneumoniae, S. aureus, S. pneumoniae* and other anaerobes (aspiration). In tropics: *Bacillus anthracis, Francisella tularensis, Yersinia pestis*
Pneumonia in the immunocompromised	HHV-1, HHV-3, HHV-5, measles Enterobacteriaceae, *H. influenzae, L. pneumophila, M. avium/intracellulare, M. tuberculosis, Nocardia* spp, *Pseudomonas* spp, *S. aureus, S. pneumoniae, Aspergillus* spp, *Cryptococcus neoformans, Mucor* spp, *Pneumocystis carinii, Strongyloides stercoralis, Toxoplasma gondii.*
Bronchiectasis and chronic obstructive airways disease	*Burkholderia cepacia* (in cystic fibrosis), *H. influenzae, Pseudomonas aeruginosa, S. aureus, Stenotrophomonas maltophilia, S. pneumoniae, Aspergillus* spp, *Candida* spp
Lung abscess and empyema	*Klebsiella pneumoniae*, anaerobes (e.g *Fusobacterium necrophorum*), *S. aureus, Streptococcus milleri, S. pneumoniae Entamoeba histolytica*

Appendix 3 Respiratory tract infections.

EXANTHEMS	
Maculopapular erythematous	Enteroviruses, HHV-4 (glandular fever), HHV-6 and 7 (exanthem subitum), HIV, measles, parvovirus (erythema infectiosum, fifth disease), rubella *Neisseria meningitidis* (septicaemia) *Salmonella typhi* *Staphylococcus aureus* (toxic shock syndrome) *Streptococcus pyogenes* (scarlet fever) *Treponema pallidum* (secondary syphilis)
Petechial purpuric	Arboviruses, adenoviruses, enteroviruses, measles (in immunocompromised) *N. meningitidis* Other Gram-negative bacterial septicemia *Rickettsia* spp
Hemorrhagic	Alphaviruses, arenaviruses, filoviruses, hantavirus, nairovirus, phlebovirus, togaviruses *Rickettsia* spp, *N. meningitidis*, *Pseudomonas aeruginosa*
Vesicular/pustalar	Enteroviruses (hand, foot and mouth disease), HHV-1 (cold sores), HHV-2 (genital herpes), HHV-3 (chickenpox and shingles), *S. aureus*, *S. pyogenes* (impetigo), monkeypox
Nodules Multiple Usually single	 Molluscum contagiosum, papillomaviruses (warts) Orthopoxvirus (cowpox, tanapox), parapoxviruses (Orf)
Kaposi's sarcoma	Kaposi's sarcoma-associated herpes virus (HHV-8)

Appendix 4 Exanthems.

GASTROINTESTINAL INFECTIONS			
	Most important	**Less common**	**Tropical or geographically limited**
Gastritis **Peptic ulceration** **Hepatitis**	*Helicobacter pylori*, *H. pylori*, Hepatitis A, B, C, D	HHV-4, HHV-5, rubella (congenital), *Brucella* spp, *Leptospira* spp, *Mycobacterium tuberculosis*, *Treponema pallidum*, *Yersinia enterocolitica*	Hepatitis E, Yellow fever, *Histoplasma capsulatum*, *Entamoeba histolytica*, *Schistosoma mansoni*
Vomiting	Norwalk agent, *Bacillus cereus* (toxin), *Staphylococcus aureus* (toxin)		–
Diarrheal disease			
Non-inflammatory	Adenovirus 40/41, astrovirus, calicivirus, Norwalk agent, rotavirus, *Aeromonas* spp, *Campylobacter* spp, Enterotoxigenic *Escherichia coli*, *Salmonella* spp, *Cryptosporidium parvum*, *Giardia lamblia*	Bredavirus, coronavirus, pestivirus, torovirus, *B. cereus*, *Clostridium perfringens* (food poisoning toxin), Enteropathogenic *E. coli*, *Plesiomonas* spp, *Vibrio parahaemolyticus*, *Blastocystis hominis*, *Enterocytozoon bieneusi* (in AIDS), *Isospora belli*,	*Trophyrema whippelii*, *Vibrio cholerae*, *Cyclospora cayetanensis*
Inflammatory	*Aeromonas* spp, *Campylobacter* spp, *Clostridium difficile*, Enteroaggregative *E. coli*, Enterohemorrhagic *E. coli*, *Salmonella* spp, *Shigella* spp	Enteroinvasive *E. coli*, *Y. enterocolitica*	*Clostridium perfringens* (pig bel), *Entamoeba histolytica*

Appendix 5   Gastrointestinal infections.

GENITOURINARY TRACT INFECTIONS	
Urinary tract	
Urethritis	*Chlamydia trachomatis, Neisseria gonorrhoeae,* HHV-2
Cystitis	*Escherichia coli* (>90%), *Staphylococcus saprophyticus,* HHV-2 (trigonitis) (Rarely *Proteus, Klebsiella, Enterococcus* spp)
Acute pyelonephritis	*E. coli* (>90%) (Rarely *Proteus, Klebsiella* spp)
Complicated urinary tract infection (by congenital defect, surgery, calculi, catheterization)	*E. coli* (30%), *Proteus* spp, *Klebsiella* spp, *Pseudomonas* spp, *Enterococcus* spp, *Candida albicans*
Genital tract	
Vulvo-vaginitis (discharge)	*Neisseria gonorrhoeae, C. trachomatis,* HHV-2, *C. albicans, Trichomonas vaginalis, Enterobius vermicularis*
Bacterial vaginosis	? *Gardnerella vaginalis,* ? *Mobiluncus* spp, ? anaerobes
Genital ulcers	HHV-2, HHV-1, *Treponema pallidum, Haemophilus ducreyi, C. trachomatis* (LGV), *Calymmatobacterium granulomatis*
Genital nodules	Human papillomaviruses, molluscum contagiosum
Ectoparasites	*Phthirius pubis, Sarcoptes scabiei*
Epididymitis	*C. trachomatis, N. gonorrhoeae, Mycobacterium tuberculosis*
Orchitis/oophoritis	Mumps
Pelvic inflammatory disease	*C. trachomatis, N. gonorrhoeae,* anaerobes *Mycoplasma hominis, Ureaplasma urealyticum M. tuberculosis, Actinomyces israelii*
Carcinoma of the cervix	Human papillomaviruses 16, 18, 33

Appendix 6 Genitourinary tract infections.

SKIN AND SOFT TISSUE INFECTIONS	
Eyes	
Blepharitis	HHV-1, HPV, molluscum contagiosum, *Staphylococcus aureus*, *Moraxella lacunata*
Conjunctivitis	Adenovirus (3, 7, 8, 19), enterovirus (70), coxsackievirus (A24), HHV-1 *Haemophilus influenzae, H. aegyptius, Streptococcus pneumoniae, Neisseria meningitidis, N. gonorrhoeae, Chlamydia trachomatis* (A–C: trachoma), *C. trachomatis* (D–K: ophthalmia neonatorum)
Keratitis	HHV-1, *S. aureus, S. pyogenes, Pseudomonas* spp, *Fusarium solani, Candida albicans, Acanthamoeba* spp
Retinitis	*Toxocara canis*, HHV-5, *Toxoplasma gondii*
Orbital cellulitis	*H. influenzae* b, *S. aureus, S. pyogenes, S. pneumoniae, Trichinella spiralis, Taenia solium*
Skin	
Carbuncle, furuncle	*S. aureus*
Vesicles	HHV-1, HHV-2, HHV-3, enteroviruses
Impetigo	*S. aureus, S. pyogenes*
Nodules	Molluscum contagiosum, human papillomavirus, cowpox, orf
Granulomas	*Mycobacterium tuberculosis, M. marinum*
Ringworm	*Microsporum, Trichophyton, Epidermophyton* spp
Intertrigo	*Candida albicans*
Tinea versicolor	*Malassezia furfur*
Infected bites	
Human	Anaerobes, *Eikenella corrodens, S. aureus, S. pyogenes*
Animal	*Capnocytophaga canimorsus, Pasteurella multocida*, anaerobes
Insect	*S. aureus, S. pyogenes*
Soft tissue	
Erysipelas	*S. pyogenes* (group A, rarely C and B)
Acute cellulitis	*S. pyogenes, H. influenzae* b, *Vibrio vulnificus, Clostridium perfringens, Bacillus anthracis, Erysipelothrix* spp, *Aeromonas hydrophila*
Necrotizing fasciitis	*S. pyogenes* Synergistic infection with *S. aureus* and anaerobes
Lymphadenitis	*Brucella* spp, *M. avium-intracellulare, M. tuberculosis, Bartonella henselae* (cat scratch disease), *S. pyogenes, Treponema pallidum*

Appendix 7 Skin and soft tissue infections.

BONE, JOINT AND MUSCLE INFECTIONS	
Bone	
Acute osteomyelitis	*Staphylococcus aureus* (95%), *Haemophilus influenzae* b, *Salmonella* spp, *Streptococcus agalactiae* (in neonates)
Chronic osteomyelitis	Anaerobes, *Brucella* spp, Enterobacteriaceae, *Mycobacterium tuberculosis*, *Pseudomonas aeruginosa*, *Staphylococcus epidermidis* (implant infection)
Joints	
Septic arthritis	*S. aureus*, *H. influenzae* b, *Streptococcus pneumoniae*, *Neisseria gonorrhoeae*, *N. meningitidis*, Enterobacteriaceae (in immunocompromised), *Brucella* spp, parvovirus, rubellavirus
Reactive arthritis (reaction to infection elsewhere)	*Campylobacter* spp, *Chlamydia trachomatis*, *N. gonorrhoeae*, *N. meningitidis*, *Salmonella* spp, *Yersinia enterocolitica*
Muscle	
Pyomyositis	*S. aureus*, *Streptococcus pyogenes*
Gas gangrene	*Clostridium perfringens*
Parasitic disease	*Toxoplasma gondii*, *cysticercosis* Hydatid disease, *Trichinella spiralis*, *Toxocara canis*, *T. cati*
Bornholm disease	Enterovirus

Appendix 8 **Bone, joint and muscle infections.**

CARDIOVASCULAR INFECTIONS	
Infective endocarditis	Viridans streptococci, *Staphylococcus epidermidis*, *Cardiobacterium hominis*, *Coxiella burnetii*, *Haemophilus aphrophilus*, *Enterococcus* spp, *Candida albicans*, *Aspergillus* spp, *Staphylococcus aureus* (acute)
Prosthetic valves	*S. epidermidis* in particular
Intravenous drug abusers	Enterobacteriaceae, *Pseudomonas aeruginosa*, *Candida* spp, in particular
Pericarditis	Coxsackie B virus *Haemophilus influenzae* b, *Streptococcus pneumoniae*, *S. pyogenes*, *S. aureus*, *Neisseria meningitidis*, *Mycobacterium tuberculosis*
Myocarditis	Coxsackie A and B, ECHO, mumps viruses *N. meningitidis*, *S. aureus*, *S. pyogenes*

Appendix 9 **Cardiovascular infections.**

FEVER OF UNKNOWN ORIGIN*

Most important		Less common
Infections (up to 40% of cases)		
Localized	Intra-abdominal abscess Subphrenic abscess Pelvic abscess Tuberculous meningitis	Perinephric abscess, splenic abscess, dental abscess, brain abscess, chronic sinusitis, chronic meningitis, chronic osteomyelitis, cholangitis, bacterial endocarditis, mastoiditis, pyelonephritis, lung abscess, hepatitis, lymphogranuloma venereum, psittacosis, Lyme disease (*Borrelia burgdorferi*)
Disseminated	HHV-4, HHV-5 HIV Miliary tuberculosis Typhoid fever Malaria	Brucellosis, relapsing fever (*Borrelia recurrentis*), rat-bite fever (*Spirillum minus*), leptospirosis, Q-fever (*Coxiella burnetii*), cat scratch disease (*Bartonella henselae*), erlichosis, *Rickettsia* spp, *Cryptococcus neoformans*, *Histoplasma capsulatum*, toxoplasmosis, toxocariasis, trypanosomiasis, Katayama fever (schistosomiasis)
Neoplasia (about 15%)	Lymphomas, hypernephroma Metastases to liver or CNS	Hepatoma, carcinoma of pancreas, atrial myxoma, neuroblastoma
Autoimmune (about 15%)	Still's disease, Giant cell arthritis	Rheumatoid arthritis, polyarteritis nodosa, systemic lupus erythematosus, Felty's syndrome, rheumatic fever
Other (10–20%)	Drug fever, Kawasaki's disease	Anhidrotic ectodermal dysplasia Diabetes insipidus Fabry's disease Factitious fever Familial dysautonomia Familial Mediterranean fever Pancreatitis Periodic fever Pulmonary embolism Serum sickness Thyrotoxicosis
Undiagnosed (10–20%)		

*Petersdorf suggests, as a definition, a minimum temperature of 38.8°C for 3 weeks with at least 1 week of intensive hospital investigation. In pediatric practice, a shorter period of fever of 1 week is often used.

Appendix 10 Fever of unknown origin.

INDEX

Note: Numbers refer to page numbers not illustration numbers.